kundalini postures
and poetry

KUNDALINI POSTURES AND POETRY

SHAKTI PARWHA KAUR KHALSA

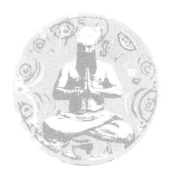

A PERIGEE BOOK

Since ancient times in India, outstanding benefits have been attributed to the practice of yoga. However, the author/compiler of this book hereby disclaims any responsibility for any such claims included herein.

There is no doubt that the practice of yoga has benefited millions of people, but this book is not intended as medical advice. Its intent is solely for information and enjoyment. The therapeutic benefits attributed come from centuries-old yogic tradition. Please consult with your physician or licensed health care practitioner before starting any exercise program.

A Perigee Book
Published by The Berkley Publishing Group
A division of Penguin Group (USA) Inc.
375 Hudson Street
New York, New York 10014

Copyright © 2003 by Shakti Parwha Kaur Khalsa
Text design by Pauline Neuwirth
Cover design by Wendy Bass
Digital imaging by Wendy Bass based on photos of the Master
A list of photo credits appears on pp.224.

First edition: May 2003

Library of Congress Cataloging-in-Publication Data
Shakti Parwha Kaur Khalsa.
Kundalini postures and poetry / compiled with rhymes by Shakti Parwha Kaur Khalsa.
p. cm.
Includes bibliographical references and index.
ISBN 0-399-52883-0 (pbk.)
1. Kundalini. I. Title.
RA781.7 .S436 2003
294.5'436—dc21   2002035511

Printed in the United States of America

10 9 8 7 6 5 4 3 2 1

To all Kundalini yoga teachers

past, present, and future.

Yoga is a science for all humanity.

It is the custodian of human grace and radiance.

It holds a great future for every human being.

It brings mental caliber for purpose and prosperity of life.

—YOGI BHAJAN

CONTENTS

ACKNOWLEDGMENTS

I WAS BLESSED to have many kind and gifted people helping me to produce this book. The process began with my search for *Yogic Therapy*, the book Yogi Bhajan cited as authentic reference to explain the postures. I contacted Satsimran Kaur who was in India, and she knew exactly where I could find it.

To get even more scientific in-depth yogic information, I taped several hours of discussion with Gurucharan Singh Khalsa, Ph.D., President of Khalsa Consultants and one of the founders of the Kundalini Research Institute. He provided wonderful insights and commentary that I adopted and adapted.

Guru Prem Singh Khalsa, whom Yogi Bhajan has given the title "Posture Master," checked the photos and provided technical tips for the "How to Do It" sections.

Without my research assistant, Dyal Kaur, I couldn't even have gotten off the ground. She referenced and cross-referenced each posture with its picture and description from various sources.

Siri Ram Kaur Khalsa made order out of chaos. An ideal Virgo, and editor of *Aquarian Times* magazine, she organized the jigsaw-puzzle pieces of material I had gathered. Her enthusiasm for the project has meant more than I can say.

My "readers," Gloria Gold (my cousin), Gobind Kaur Khalsa, Guru Raj Kaur Khalsa, Satya Kaur Khalsa, Harijot Kaur Khalsa, Ek Ong Kar Kaur Khalsa, and Ted Garon (my brother), each made valuable (and necessary) corrections, suggestions, and comments on the first draft. Their encouragement has been heartwarming. What a family!

God and Guru really came through when I was searching for a graphic designer. Mandy Hurwitz, a yoga student recently arrived from South Africa, appeared at Yoga West in Los Angeles, where I teach. She perfectly captured the feeling and the intention of this book. And what a delight she was to work with!

Seva Kaur Khalsa (currently a designer for KIIT Inc.) generously shared her keen artist's eye and her suggestions enhanced the design process.

In the search for a literary agent to represent this work, several fellow authors kindly gave me the names of their agents. Thank you to Dr. Dharma Singh Khalsa, Gurumukh Kaur Khalsa, and Gloria Gold. It was Shakta Kaur Khalsa's agent, Jeff Herman, who saw the potential in this book, and thanks to his efforts, we are in print.

Special accolades to my editor, Sheila Curry Oakes, and her staff at Perigee Books who are bountifully helpful, beautifully patient, and blissfully easy to work with.

Gurucharan Singh Khalsa, Ph.D., is an eminent Lecturer, Psychologist, Teacher and originator of the *Breath-Walk* seminars. He is co-author of Yogi Bhajan's *The Mind Book* and *The Masters Touch.*

Guru Prem Singh Khalsa has worked as a Movement and Postural Therapist at the Khalsa Medical Clinic in Beverly Hills for over twenty years. He is a KRI Certified Kundalini Yoga Teacher trainer.

FOREWORD

Dear Reader,

SOME BOOKS YOU read, some books you study; this book you can savor. You can nibble at it a section at a time or devour the whole thing in a single sitting. It will be a pleasure either way.

Shakti's secret is her blend of reason and rhyme on every page. It is that same blend that leads us to feel life at its best. Reason helps us to live within the universal laws of matter. Rhyme helps us to live within the universal laws of spirit. With reason we are effective. With rhyme we express the poetry of our heart so we feel meaningful and real.

To embody this blend of reason and rhyme into each moment of our life, into each breath, takes a refined consciousness and great self-mastery. That capacity comes from the touch of a master who has attained that inner balance and who shares it through his or her presence, teaching, and example. Yogi Bhajan's masterful touch inspired Shakti Parwha to imbue this collection of photos and postures with gratitude, love, and insight. She was his first student in the West and continues to teach us all.

As you read the first few pages it is clear that a posture is not just a stance. A posture adds flexibility to awareness and not just to muscle and ligament.

Taking a stance is half of taking a posture. A stance is when we position our body with precision and reason. We stand according to the laws of gravity, geometry, and anatomy. We position ourselves to prepare to act.

The other half of taking a posture requires poetry. Poetry goes beyond the laws of physics, forces, and geometry to capture the subtlety and richness that defines us as human beings. Poetry opens our feelings. It is all about proportions, like chords in music and ratios in numbers. Poetry uses silence and sound, words and tone, repetition and metaphors to evoke our awareness. To make us present. To change us deeply as we awaken inner attitudes and possibilities.

For a Kundalini yogi, posture is stance and awareness, reason and rhyme, geometry and poetry. It is when body, mind, spirit, and self all harmonize.

When I saw what Shakti Parwha Kaur had done, I smiled so hard I almost broke my face. As a director of teacher training, I have shelves of yoga books filled with postures. Page after page, book after book the same descriptions are repeated with precise anatomical terms and ever leaner models.

This book is different. The posture this book takes is one of a kind. Its simplicity adds depth. Its devotion reveals the inner beauty that all yoga strives for.

The touch of the Master is everywhere in these pages. The photo album approach is personal, historical, and unique. She inspires us in an ancient way: modeling a master. These are actual photos of a master of Kundalini Yoga doing the practice. We can look and learn, see and do.

Shakti inspires us in a modern way—her rhymes convey the attitudes that turn stances into postures. And her humor makes information and wisdom accessible and effortless to absorb.

This book is now one of the first assignments my students read to explore a new relationship to their body through posture.

Who should read this book? Yoga students, of course. And anyone who wants to think of his or her body differently. In our culture we struggle mightily with the image of our body and our feelings toward it. This album reminds us of the sacred dimension to our body. And it is for anyone curious about what they have heard about yoga and who wants a first look, peppered with wisdom, quotations, and humor.

Enjoy the journey.

—GURUCHARAN SINGH KHALSA, PH.D.,
director of training, Kundalini Research Institute

xiv

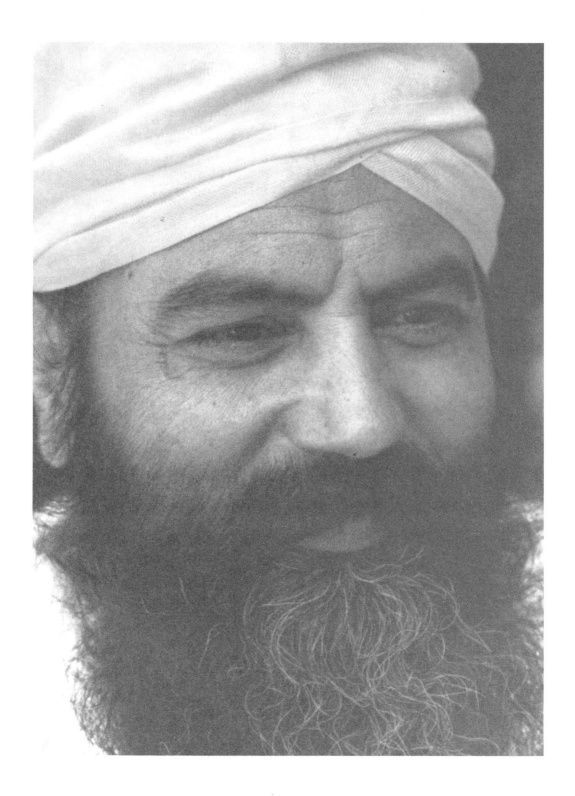

A Special Note for Women During Menstruation and Pregnancy

NO INVERTED postures, no Breath of Fire, no postures lying on the stomach; no application of the lower locks (Neck Lock is okay, but not Mul Bandh). No cold showers during entire menstrual period. Women between four and seven months pregnant can take a short cold shower (no more than three minutes) but no cold showers after the seventh month of pregnancy and not until forty days after the birth.

1

FRAMING THE PHOTOS

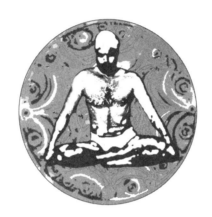

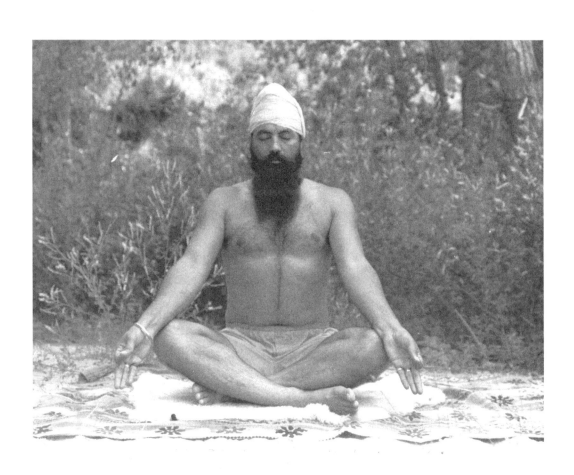

Framing the Photos

(HOW THIS BOOK CAME INTO BEING)

This book was commissioned by the Master himself
When I showed him these photos I'd kept on a shelf
More than thirty years since he gave the album to me
Shortly after he arrived from across the sea.

He said, "Make the photos into a book,
And explain the postures in rhyme."
Though I thought, "Oh, no!" — what I said was, "Yes, sir."
(That's what you do when you have a teacher like mine!)

Actually he said "poetry" but I wouldn't presume
To call these verses poetry, though I trust that they will scan,
I hope they meet with your approval—
I've done the best I can.

I researched the texts from India he recommended,
Trying to make things clear
Describing the benefits of the postures
That Yogi Bhajan demonstrates here.

It's not intended as a yoga manual
It's a keepsake for generations to come:
Pictures of the Master of Kundalini Yoga
Showing what he has done.

Note: Most of the photos in this book were taken in India when Yogi Bhajan was about thirty-nine. The other posture photos were taken in New Mexico by Lisa Law in 1981, when he was fifty-two.

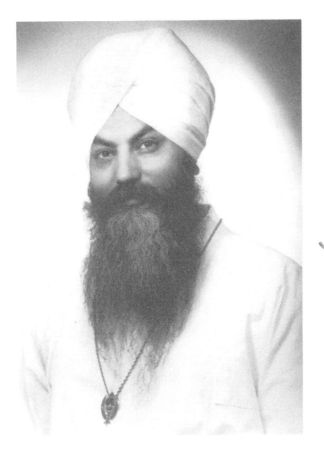

THROUGHOUT RECORDED history, there have been a rare few spiritual giants whose lives, teachings, and very presence on the planet have accelerated the progress of millions of souls. Such a master is my spiritual teacher, Yogi Bhajan. He has set the blueprint for what it means to be a true and sacred spiritual teacher for this New Age, the Age of Aquarius.

In November 1991 we entered into a twenty-one-year cusp period (divided into three seven-year increments) leading into the actual New Age, the Age of Aquarius. We are leaving the Piscean Age. This shift in major astrological eras is marked by major changes in the world and a lot of chaos. Human consciousness is changing. Political, social, economic, religious—all aspects of human interaction (and inner awareness) are shifting. Group consciousness—people working together—has to manifest.

Born in India on August 26, 1929, Yogi Bhajan mastered Kundalini Yoga at the age of sixteen. A career in government service sent him on extensive travels throughout India. He made it a point to meet and learn from every yoga master he could find.

He tells how he saw Westerners arriving in New Delhi with high spiritual hopes and lots of money in their pockets. He watched them leave India with empty pockets and not much spiritual enlightenment to show for their efforts. This betrayal of their aspiration affected him deeply.

When he arrived in the United States in late 1968, Yogi Bhajan stated his mission quite clearly: "I have come to create teachers, not to gather disciples." Such a master is not a philosopher or a preacher. He is a transmitter of the same mastery that he has achieved.

He was the first person who ever dared to teach Kundalini Yoga openly to the public. In 1969 he established the 3HO Foundation ("3HO" stands for "Healthy, Happy, Holy Organization") to spread the teachings of Kundalini Yoga. He is the Mahan Tantric, the only living master of White Tantric Yoga, a powerful group meditation technique that releases subconscious blocks. He generously shares the experience of this transformational yoga through day-long meditation courses.

His belief that "there is no power greater than the power of prayer" has resulted in the International Peace Prayer Day Music Celebration held every year in the Jemez Mountains of New Mexico, bringing people of all faiths together to pray for peace.

Today, in his early seventies, Yogi Bhajan is still traveling, lecturing, guiding, and teaching wherever he goes. As the chief religious and administrative authority for the Sikh religion in the Western Hemisphere, he holds the ministerial title of Siri Singh Sahib of Sikh Dharma.

His motto is, If you can't see God in all, you can't see God at all.

Yogi Bhajan, Teacher of Teachers

❈

Traditionally taught in secrecy, to proven devotees only,
Yogi Bhajan broke the taboo, when he dared teach Kundalini Yoga openly.
He took his life in his hands, and on the altar of truth
Shared what he knew, to rescue the youth.

It was the sixties, times had changed, the Aquarian Age had dawned.
His divine wisdom foretold the chaos to come.
He came to train teachers, healers to be,
By the grace of Guru Ram Das, servants of humanity.

"Don't love me, love my teachings instead."
"You are the grace of God," to the women, he said.
"It's not the life that matters, it's the courage you bring."
We quoted his sayings—they became songs that we sing.
"Faith moves mountains, otherwise even stones are heavy for a man."
"Doing is believing"—"Take a cold shower in the morning—yes you can!"

"Yogic tidbits" he shared with us,
Habits of living without any fuss:
How to wake up in the morning, how to go to sleep at night;
He taught us a graceful way of living
In which "the greatest happiness comes from giving."

He gave us gems of sacred wisdom, scattered them far and wide,
Sharing everything he had to offer, nothing to hide.

6

He didn't ask for perfection, he told us to "Look inside,
Find the real You in you, and put all your fears aside."

Then, "Become ten times greater than me!"
Came the provocative challenge from Yogiji.
How could students improve upon mastery that never fails?
"Well," we thought, "we can try to fill in some details,
To refine and perfect, to polish and shine
Our physical bodies as well as our minds."

And so under his guidance we became more precise,
Researching material that could give us advice.
Some became experts in posture correction;
Teachers branched out in many directions.
Books were written and videos made
To ensure Kundalini Yoga will never fade.

The yogi is one who has a union with his supreme consciousness.

If flexibility of the body is the only yoga,

then clowns in the Circus are the best yogis.

—Yogi Bhajan

Purpose of Yoga

❧

Yoga is great for gaining flexibility and physical health all around;
But the real purpose of yoga is far more profound.
"Yoga" means to yoke (or unite) your individual consciousness
    with the universal Self—
This "divine union" is the ultimate goal of all human existence,
    not fame, not power, not wealth.

But by all means (righteous, of course!), succeed in your earthly pursuits.
Make the most of this human experience—but don't forget your roots:
All things come from God and all things, including you, shall return
When the lessons for which your soul incarnated have been learned.
Death is just a "going Home," so when consciously, yogically done,
You can leave the Earth plane fearlessly, for liberation you have won.

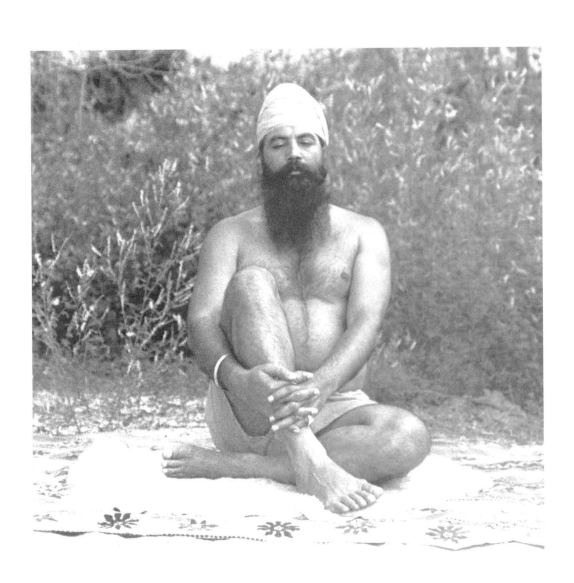

Liberation

❀

When you die, your Soul Body leaves in the Subtle Body,[1]
like a space capsule blasting toward the ethers blue.
Yoga classes are like NASA, preparing for the journey Home,
when your turn as space traveler is due.

Get used to the higher realms through meditation,
    talk to your soul through prayer,
That's the way to ensure a safe and smooth journey there.

You are a divine Being of Light, given a human form on Earth.
To experience His creation through you, God gave you this physical birth.
So chant SAT NAM and WAHE GURU plus other mantras too,
To clear away the screen of illusion, the maya that hides the real You from you.
Practice Kundalini Yoga, meditate and chant in the early morning hours
Make friends with your inner Truth, that immortal Self, which is always yours.

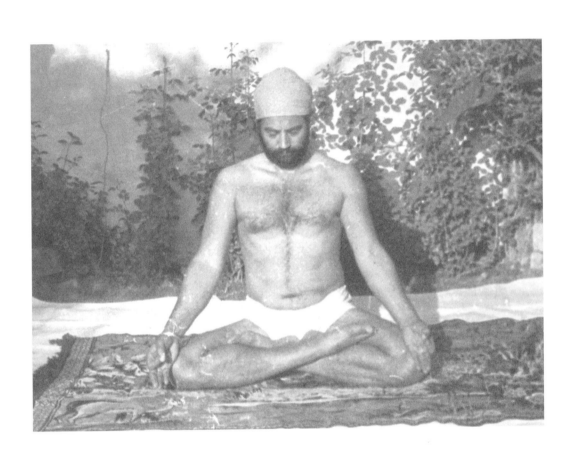

Supermodels with Stunning Dimensions

❈

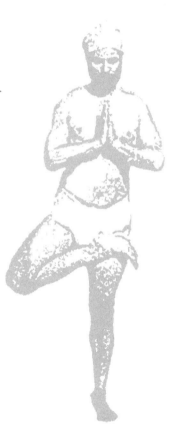

Supermodels with stunning dimensions (still in their teens)
Or perfectly flexible athletes (in your dreams!):
These are the people we usually see in the books
Making us aspire to such wonderful looks.
We sigh and we groan, and we get body tucks,
But we're missing the point when we spend all those bucks.

Real beauty lies within—it's not just a platitude.
Discover the enchantment of the body—it's an inner attitude.
The whole is greater than the sum of its parts;
Postures combined with breath and motion form this art.

Using outer postures to transform the inner,
Whether you're a seasoned practitioner or just a beginner,
You have the power to transform your life
And you don't need a hypodermic, you don't need a knife!

Perfect harmony between body and mind,
Happiness and health you're sure to find.
Balance and beauty come from within—
Kundalini Yoga is the place to begin.

THE GIFT OF YOGA

Yogis have known for centuries how to achieve radiant beauty and power—using the body and the mind. These yogic techniques come from a tradition that never lost the keys to unlocking the body's mystery and the potential of the human soul. It is this enchantment of the body that we really seek, whether we know it or not.

This enchantment is already in each and every one of us, waiting to be experienced, just as our inner radiance is waiting patiently to be released. Every single human being has this great potential locked inside.

Yogi Bhajan is the teacher who openly shared with us the keys to unlocking the enchantment of the body. He is living proof that a person who lives in the world, dealing with the same day-to-day situations that confront all of us, can not only experience the wonder and joy of Kundalini Yoga, but even master it!

Yogi Bhajan did not become a master by achieving physical perfection; he became a master by conquering his mind, opening his heart, and merging with his highest spirit.

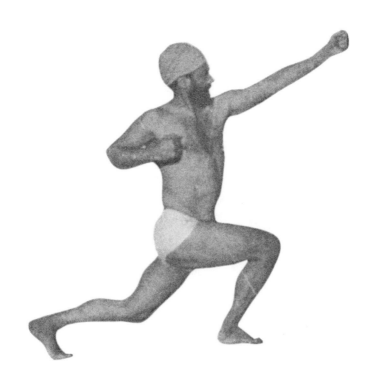

"Postures are the alphabet of communication to the body, and when we do certain postures in specified sequence, we create poetry in motion. The outer postures trigger a release of the tension patterns which I will call 'inner postures' that have been held in the subconscious. These patterns of tension in the subconscious develop as we grow up and are the hidden cause of much of our suffering. They are the blocks that prevent us from changing the behavioral habits that bring us pain.

"Yogi Bhajan didn't simply teach us postures, he taught us kriyas. A kriya is literally defined as a 'completed action.' It is the dynamic use of posture or a sequence of postures, combined with a breathing pattern, a sound current, and motion. Kundalini Yoga is the fountainhead of knowledge of these powerful kriyas, of which there are thousands. (A posture is like a petal on a flower—its beauty and power are only understood as part of a full bloom: the kriya.)

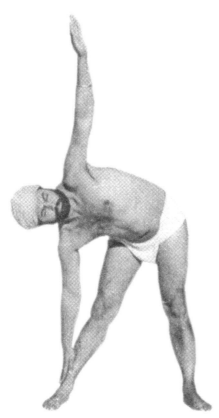

Everyone knows about body language. It's universal. The yogis took this a step further by discovering, and then revealing, the specific postures of the body that communicate to the inner self, perfecting and balancing with the outer self. There are many facets to this conversation between the inner and the outer."[2]

Kundalini Yoga

If change makes you insecure, better take care—
Kundalini Yoga will make you . . . aware.
You won't be the same when you leave the cocoon;
This transformation takes place very soon.
You'll discover your power, beauty, and grace
As kundalini rises, Destiny comes face to face.

Nothing is forced, kundalini is allowed to rise
When you practice the teachings, you'll be surprised
How quickly you discover your identity is divine
SAT NAM[3] becomes your motto (repeat it anytime).

Mastery of Self is the name of the game
So you enjoy your life; understand why you came
To visit planet Earth and your soul took birth.
Time has come to recognize your worth:
You are a spiritual being in human form
Living consciously should be your norm.

And when the job you came for is done
You'll leave your body behind and return Home to the One
Who gave you the Earth as playground and school
To enjoy and to learn, governed by cosmic rules.
Yes, "As you sow, so shall you reap"—
This Law of Karma we all must keep

Until we break the cycle and become consciously aware.
Kundalini Yoga, by the grace of the Guru, will take us there.
In the process, it will tune up your nerves
And make your glands secrete
But Kundalini Yoga
Performs an even greater feat:

Opening your third eye, your intuition becomes strong,
In your decisions you won't go wrong;
Wisely using your mind and emotions too,
Instead of having them use you!

The whole is greater than the sum of its parts
We learn in Kundalini Yoga right from the start.
Asanas are basic, pranayam is fine,
Plus mudras and mantra in kriyas combine
With powerful effect on glands, organs, and nerves;
In a very short time, kriyas awaken energy reserves.

You don't have to be perfect in flexibility or pose
Just do your best—and remember your ONG NAMO'S.

ONG NAMO GURU DEV NAMO[+]
invokes the Masters who guide this path
Each a link in the golden chain from the past
Where yoga was born as a tool for mankind
To liberate us from traveling blind.

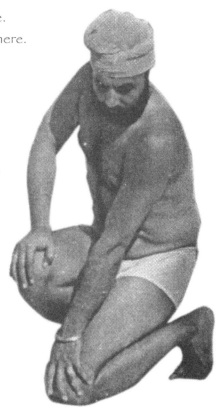

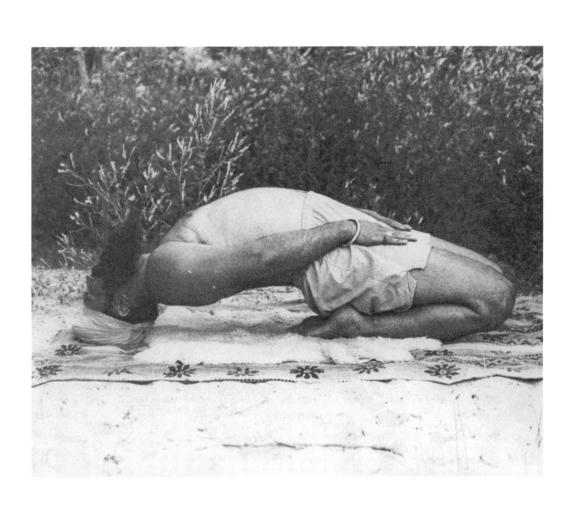

Asanas and Patanjali

❧

In the beginning Yogi Bhajan knew we were raw
But our potential and the future were what he saw.
He made yoga so easy, we couldn't resist,
On perfect posture he didn't insist.
Emphasis on Asanas could come later on
When aspiration and transformation of character had begun.
First he taught us to breathe and to chant God's name,
Do Sadhana every morning, so we'd never be the same.
Now it's three decades later, and we strive with yogic grace
To deal with unruly arms and legs, put them in their proper place.
You see, Asanas (the postures) are step number three
In the well-ordered sequence laid out by Patanjali.

Patanjali said:
You start with the Yams and the Niyams, the dont's and the do's:
Thoughts, words, and actions to consciously choose
To lay the foundation for human success.
Then—and only then—begin Asanas, if you want happiness.
Perfecting each posture brings maximum gain
When incorporated into heart and brain.
Pranayam and Pratyahar—
     yogic breathing and mind control—will take you far
Toward concentration and meditation, Dharana and Dhyan:
Next steps on the path you've started upon.

PERFECT AND CORRECT

There is "perfect" posture, and there is "correct" posture. Perfection is not attainable by everyone. Hatha yogis sit in caves or on top of mountains for days and weeks and months at a time to perfect their postures. We, on the other hand, have other things that demand our time. We have not given up all of our possessions and renounced the world. We lead busy, active, demanding lives, with many responsibilities to fulfill. Fortunately, it doesn't take long to experience noticeable results from practicing Kundalini Yoga a few minutes a day. It is tailor-made for people with homes and families and careers. Simply by doing some of the classic yoga postures correctly, and in a prescribed sequence, with the added impact of mantra and pranayam, we get positive results from Kundalini Yoga, the Yoga of Awareness.

Almost anyone can do Kundalini Yoga exercises correctly. Find a 3HO Yoga Center (www.3ho.org; yoginfo@3ho.org) and take some classes; then judge for yourself. "Doing is believing."[5] Even if, like me, you're not the most flexible person in the world, you will still benefit. Truly, it is one's personal effort that brings results.

What results are we looking for? Peace of mind, expanded awareness, increased capability in all areas of our lives, and the ability to concentrate and stay focused and calm, no matter what stressful situation confronts us.

It is your birthright to be healthy, happy, and holy, and Kundalini Yoga is a practical and proven method to help you claim that birthright.

Perfection

Perfection is rare on this planet
Though we may strive to achieve it.
To some fortunate souls, near perfection is granted,
They are certainly blessed to receive it.

In this world of imperfection, let us aim for the ideal
By doing things correctly, for that is doable and real.

All human beings have one thing in common. The breath of life is one

common thing. . . . If there is anything divine in you, it's your breath.

Every inhalation you receive is a reaffirmation

of God's presence in you.

— YOGI BHAJAN

2

BREATH OF LIFE

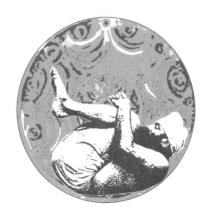

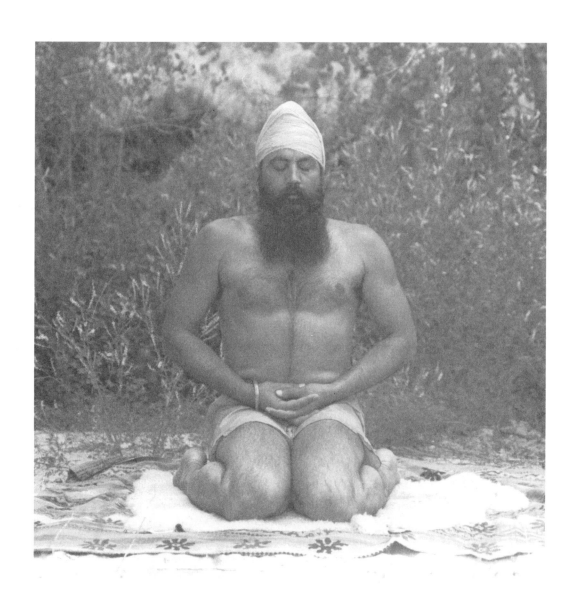

Breath of Life: Prana

❧

Breath of life is your life, in fact it has been said:
"Folks, if you don't get your next inhalation,
You're dead."

No fooling, no joke, the gift of life we receive
With every inhalation, only so long as God wants us to breathe.

It's not the air we breathe that keeps us alive
The prana each inhalation brings is the reason we survive.
That force, that Intelligence, the one Creator,
   God, bestows life upon each creature
So God can experience His creation, enjoy each event and every feature.

To enhance the quality of life, to work directly with its Source,
Yogis developed pranayam, the science of breathing—consciously, of course!

Long Deep Breathing

❦

Inhale DEEP, fill the abdomen first, then bring prana into chest and neck;
Breathing long and deep only through the nose; with your higher Self connect.

In Kundalini Yoga, all breathing is through the nose, unless otherwise instructed.
You have two nostrils designed for this purpose; that's how you were constructed.

The master architect who designed the human bodies (of which you each have ten)[1]
Made your state of mind dependent upon your rate of breathing. So then
The slower you breathe, the calmer you get, as your mind slows down, too.
"The mind follows the breath, the body follows the mind."
This fact can be useful to you.

Meditation on the Breath

If you're under stress, upset or afraid,
Meditate on your breath, worries will fade.
With eyes closed, watch it flow in and watch it flow out.
Remember Who is breathing in you (that's what life is all about).

Inhale think SAT, exhale think NAM,
As your breath slows down, your mind becomes calm.
("Nam" is identity, yours and mine
"Sat" means truth, beyond space and time.)

Receive each inhalation gratefully, it's a gift from your Creator.
An "attitude of gratitude"—a powerful tool—makes you, as a human being, even
   greater!

Breathing slower than eight times a minute automatically makes your pituitary secrete.
   Increases the flow of intuition through your sixth Chakra[2]—
Awareness becomes more complete.
Breathe less than four times a minute, you're in a meditative state.
Breath of Fire helps increase lung capacity so you can handle this pace
 (try doing it with a smile on your face!).
Breath of Fire seems fast, but it counts as only one breath—from beginning to end;
It automatically slows your rate of breathing, my friend.

   NOTE: Always breathe only through the nose unless otherwise instructed.

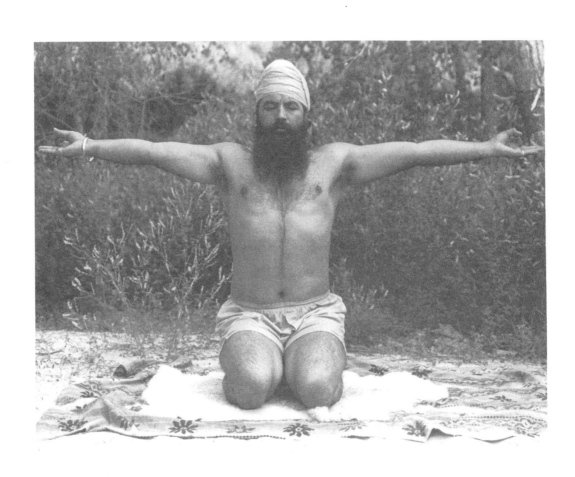

Breath of Fire

Kindly imagine, if you will
Twenty-six steam engines chugging uphill.
The soundtrack for this adventure, your breathing provides,
See those engines take the hill in stride!
Powerful, rapid breathing through the nose,
Breath of Fire is the soundtrack I propose.
Inhale and exhale of equal proportion
To claim wonderful benefits is no distortion.
Breath of Fire strengthens your seventy-two thousand nerves and expands your
    lungs,
Purifies the bloodstream, makes you feel energetic and young!
Use your navel as the point of power in you
Pull it in as you exhale (and the diaphragm too).
Inhale is easy, no stress, no strain,
Breath of Fire should cause no pain.
Keep the rhythm steady, chest slightly lifted, not in motion.
120 to 180 breaths per minute, practice with devotion:
    Listen to the sound your breathing makes,
    A couple of minutes is all it takes,
    Then relax, the engines have put on their brakes.

REASON

A dramatic name for a dramatic breathing pattern, the Breath of Fire pranayam is
used in many different postures in Kundalini Yoga kriyas. It will completely readjust
your nervous system and give you nerves of steel.

The benefits of only one to three minutes of Breath of Fire include:

- ❀ Alertness, energy, and strength
- ❀ Expanded lung capacity and vital breath
- ❀ Expulsion of toxins from the lung tissues
- ❀ Cleared mucus membranes
- ❀ Balanced autonomic nervous system
- ❀ Loss of addictive impulses

How to do It

THE BREATH is simple: rapid breathing through the nose unless otherwise specified. Keep the length of the inhale and the exhale completely equal. Rhythm is more important than speed. Your breathing should be continuous and very smooth; your nostrils should remain relaxed and not squeezed shut by your breathing.

To exhale doing Breath of Fire, expel the air by pressing your navel point in and up as you contract your diaphragm.

The inhale happens when you relax your diaphragm so that it extends downward. That allows your breath to come in naturally with little effort. Your chest should stay relaxed and slightly lifted throughout the breathing cycle. Remember to keep the ratio completely equal.

IT JUST TAKES a bit of practice so you can keep the cadence steady. An erratic rhythm will be irritating and risks leading to an oxygen imbalance.

When the ratio is equal, your breath gains a momentum and becomes easy. You will find yourself becoming alert, energized, and relaxed at the same time. Keep your upper chest slightly lifted.

When perfected, the rate should be 120 to 180 cycles per minute. A cycle is one inhalation and one exhalation. This is pretty fast!

Some people work too hard at this. If you're not sure if you're doing it right, put one hand on your upper chest and the other hand between your solar plexus and your navel point. The upper hand on your chest should remain still while you do Breath of Fire. The power comes from below. Relax your face, relax your shoulders, and just breathe. Your lower palm should feel the upper abdomen near your solar plexus pulsating with your breath. If you now move your lower hand beneath your navel point, you will find that almost no movement occurs. Breath of Fire is not a lower belly pump (that would be a different technique, called Bellows Breath).

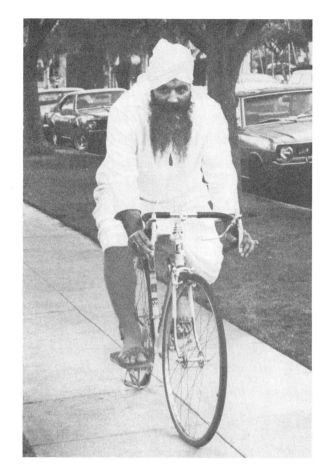

Don't forget Breath of Fire is a purifying breath. It helps to flush out the toxins in your bloodstream, so when you first do it, it can make you feel slightly giddy. Yogic wisdom tells us to use common sense when developing any new physical skill, especially breathing techniques. So of course take it slowly while you're learning. You can start by practicing Breath of Fire for just a few minutes in thirty-second segments, taking a few long deep breaths in between. Then increase to forty-five seconds—building up to one or two minutes. Later you'll be able to do Breath of Fire much longer without a break.

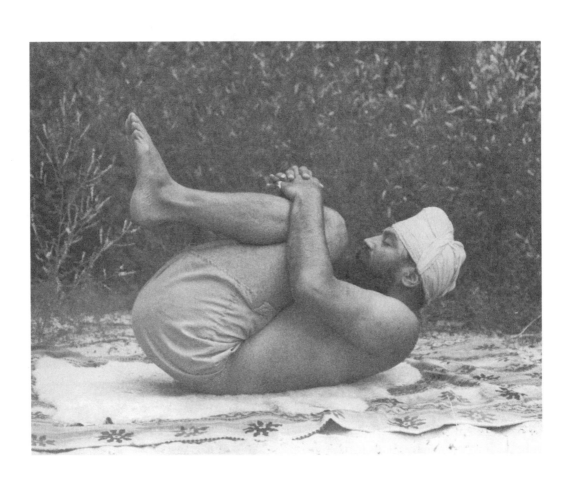

Nerves That Serve

❦

Neatly attached to our twenty-six vertebrae
are seventy-two thousand nerves with which we have to deal
Is it any wonder that so often we feel
Worn to a frazzle, stretched out so taut
That we're ready to scream? Well, that's why we ought
To strengthen our nerves and keep a supple spine
So we can remain centered; not only willing,
    but able, to toe an emotional line.
When you build extra insulation in your circuitry
    by doing Breath of Fire
Your nerves support an unflappable nature
    that people respect and admire.

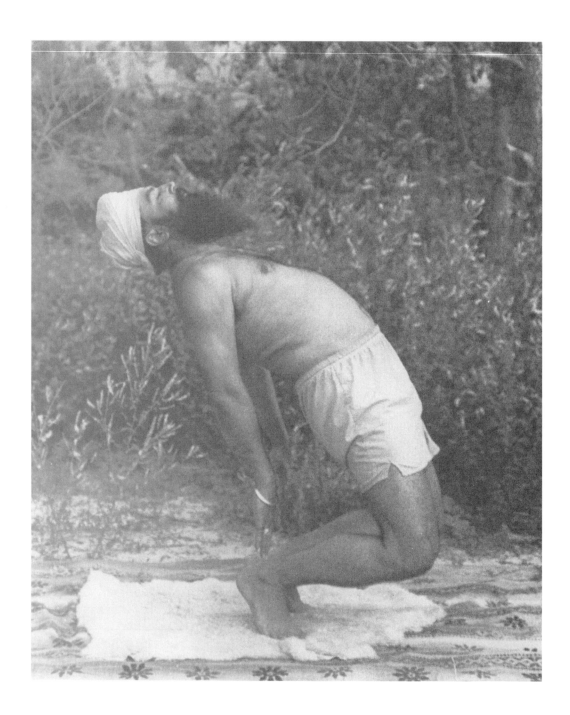

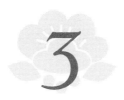

3

DAY BY DAY
IN THE CORRECT WAY

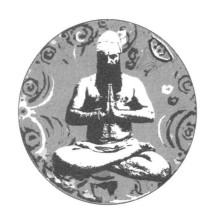

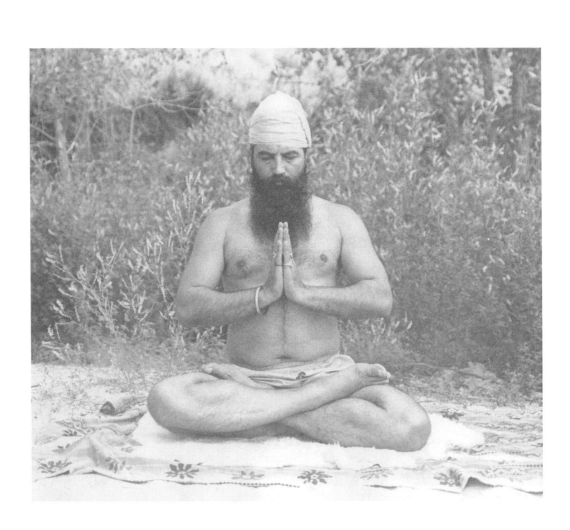

Prayer Pose: Beauty and Power

✿

For any endeavor if you want to succeed
Concentration is what you need.
Banish random thoughts from a scattered mind,
Center yourself with Prayer Pose and find
It doesn't just look "holy," it really brings peace,
Your creativity and receptivity it's sure to release.
Baking a cake or writing a sonnet—
Everything goes better when you concentrate on it.
No interruption or distraction can make you disjointed,
Practice Prayer Pose, keep your focus, and stay one-pointed.

THE INNER MAGIC OF PRAYER POSE

Prayer Pose is seen in every spiritual tradition. It is a posture of supplication. It lets us listen. It brings out an inner beauty that comes from our firm entwinement with that which is divine in our nature. . . . This mudra (hand and arm position) embodies the experience of balance and creates a seed which, when cultivated, grows into beauty, and ultimately into graceful actions.

The appreciation of beauty is an instinct deep inside us. Some of humankind's greatest accomplishments have been motivated by this innate appreciation of beauty. Mathematicians use it just as much as artists and musicians and, of course, lovers! "The inner fountain source of beauty is balance. When we see balance in a posture or a structure, we are enchanted. When we are able to feel balance inside ourselves, we act with grace and consciousness."[1]

The nerve endings in the palms of the hands connect with the two hemispheres of the brain, so pressing the two palms firmly together brings the two hemispheres of the brain into balance. This helps concentration, enabling us to be one-pointed and focused. As we apply pressure with the sides of the hands at the sternum, we stimulate a nerve ending the yogis call the "mind nerve." This nerve goes up to the brain. Thus Prayer Pose positions us physically and emotionally to focus, not only in our meditation, but in all areas of our daily lives; by training our minds to maintain concentration.

How to do It

WE START each class or practice session in Kundalini Yoga by sitting cross-legged in Easy Pose (Sukhasan) with our hands folded in the mudra called Prayer Pose. It is in this position that we chant ONG NAMO GURU DEV NAMO (see page 180) to connect with our inner teacher, as well as to receive the help and guidance of the saints and masters who have preceded us on this path. "First create physical balance by sitting cross-legged in Easy Pose (Sukhasan). Sit with your spine erect but at ease. Fold your legs to create a firm symmetric foundation. Pull your chin in slightly to release tension in the neck, and allow your head to perch fluidly on the spine. The palms of your hands are pressed firmly together, touching your chest at the sternum for equilibrium. . . . Let your breath gradually slow down and deepen, bringing a feeling of peace, contentment, and gratitude for the gift of life you receive with each inhalation."[2]

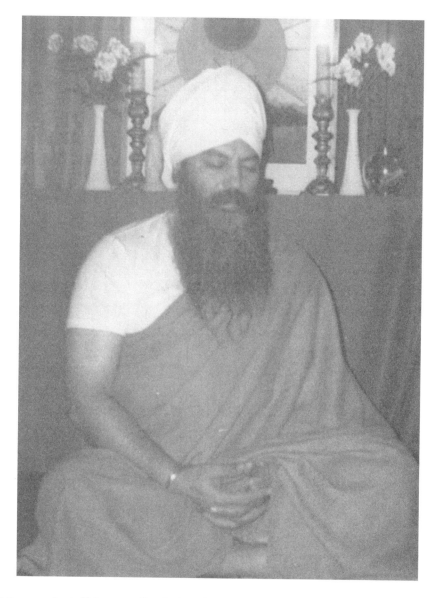

"Prayer is talking to God. Meditating is letting God talk to you."

—Yogi Bhajan

REASON

"In the center of the stomach, the navel center reposes in the circle known as Manipura. Between the navel and the last bone of the spinal column is the navel center, shaped like a bird's egg. This encloses within itself the starting points of seventy-two thousand nerves, of which seventy-two are vital. Of these, again, ten are the most important. In order to have proper control over these ten nerves, one has to take special pains."[3]

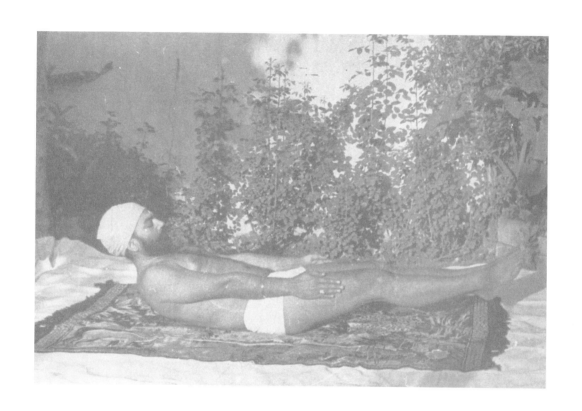

Stretch Pose

(HASTPADASANA)

Start your day the yogic way: adjust your navel while still in bed,
Up six to twelve inches bring your heels, your shoulders, and your head.
Lower back stays down flat, hands facing each other at each side
Like a sentry at Buckingham Palace—except your smile don't hide.

Stretch Pose adjusts your navel, makes your reproductive glands strong
Do it at least once a day—I'm not steering you wrong.
All seventy-two thousand nerves at your navel converge, the Upanishads supply
   the quote,
Read on, gentle reader, see what the ancient sages wrote:

> Before yoga became popular in the West, we used to make jokes about yogis
> "contemplating their navels." We thought it was funny. Well, the fact is,
> according to yogic science, the navel center is the most important position
> in the human system!

REASON

The navel center is the central control that monitors the seventy-two thousand
nerves and arteries in the entire body and makes sure they do their jobs correctly.
No matter what we do to prevent disease, no matter how much exercise we do, and
how carefully we eat, the yogis say if the navel center is defective, all the efforts we
make to remain healthy will be a waste of time and energy!

How Does the Navel Get Displaced?

Lifting weights the wrong way or falling from a height can dislodge your navel. If you put too much weight on one foot, or if one side of your body gets hit really hard, that blow can affect your navel center. When the navel gets dislodged from its correct position, this displacement invites all kinds of illnesses, many of which doctors can't diagnose.

Some of the diseases said by the yogis to come from a displaced navel are constipation, acidity, and even diseases of the heart. Loose bowel movements, colic pain, bad dreams(!), and women's monthly irregularities are other symptoms of a displaced navel.

By the way, constipation is a major cause of illness. The medical tradition of Ayurveda maintains that "unclean bowels are the breeding ground of all diseases."[4]

Stretch Pose Helps to Adjust the Navel

No wonder we are told to do Stretch Pose every morning, even before getting out of bed! (See "Morning and Night, Do It Right," page 186.) You'll find Stretch Pose included in many Kundalini Yoga kriyas.

The navel point is your life point. You can feel a pulsation at your navel by putting all five fingertips of one hand gently at the belly button while you are lying on your back. This pulsation is like the beat of your heart. When the soul is getting ready to leave the body (the condition we call "death"), even before the heart stops beating the pulsation at the navel stops.

How to do It

"TURN YOUR hips under. Lengthen the back of your neck by applying the neck lock (pull your chin in). Try to keep your lower back pressed down. You don't want to be able to see any daylight showing through. One way to keep the lower back down is to start the position by lifting the legs higher, and then lowering them down to the twelve-inch (or six-inch) height, while you keep the back down by pulling your navel down toward the floor".[5]

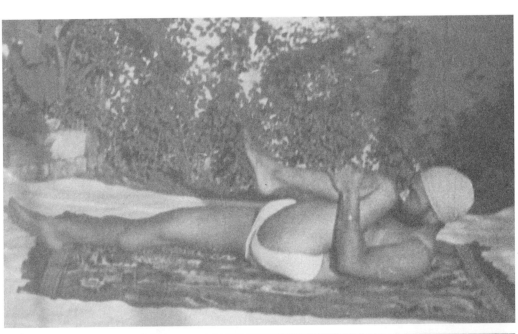

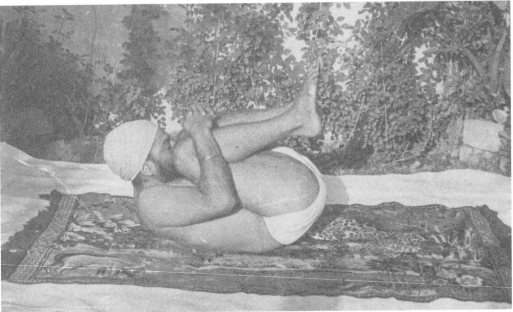

Powan Muktasana

"GAS" POSE

Start off slowly, press one knee to your chest,
Hold a few seconds and then you can rest.
Repeat on the other side five to ten seconds each time
Then inhale, head up, nose pressed into knees
Which you hug with your arms and give a good squeeze.
Removes indigestion and acidity (no pill required)
Daily practice produces a flat belly to be admired.
It's part of our 3HO yogic wake-up routine
Preceded by Stretch Pose in bed makes your day superkeen.

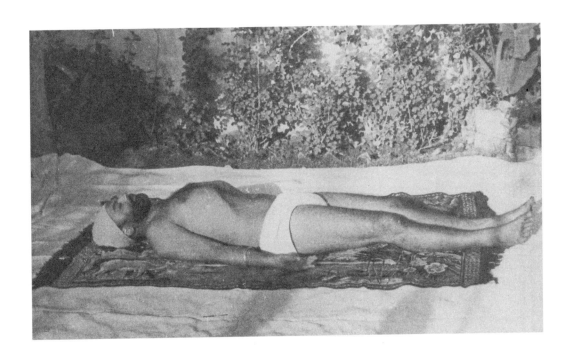

The greatest art of life is to be relaxed against all calamities

—YOGI BHAJAN

Corpse Pose: Dead While Yet Alive

SHAVASANA

Stress is a killer, so yogis learn to relax
You'll live longer when you breathe slower,
That's a fact.

When you feel worn out, overworked, and tired
Corpse Pose gets rid of the tension, you don't have to be wired!
You can live calmly in the midst of the storm,
Claim your birthright to be
Healthy, happy, holy, and calm.

Best relaxation:
Friend of blood pressure and heart patients too,
Fifteen minutes in Corpse Pose and you will renew.
Ideal repose for body and mind—
Get by on less sleep—a bonus-extra you'll find.

REASON

The yogis know that true relaxation is essential for our health and well-being. It is said that you can actually heal yourself through complete yogic relaxation. "When you are at ease, there's no dis-ease."[6]

Through deep relaxation, we can access a natural state of inner peace and tranquility. When we become still enough, our body and mind achieve their natural balance. That is the inner magic of Corpse Pose.

There is an art to achieving deep relaxation. To reach that totally calm and peaceful innermost being, we have to become dead still, like a corpse! It takes conscious care and understanding to practice this seemingly simple and effortless posture correctly.

Note: In the yogic teachings, the practice of Corpse Pose is particularly recommended for heart disease or blood pressure patients. Beyond its immediate physical benefits, it has also been recorded that many yogis have entered into the realms of higher consciousness (Yoga Nidra Trance, Samadhi) while in Corpse Pose.[7]

SUBSTITUTE FOR SLEEP

Suppose you are so tired that your nerves are telling you to sleep, but you have to stay awake. Maybe you need to study for an exam. Or you're at work and you absolutely must stay alert. What can you do? Drink black coffee? Take a pill? Please don't! There's a better solution. Take a few minutes to totally relax in Corpse Pose. Yogic texts say that if well mastered, Corpse Pose can substitute for sleep.

Almost every Kundalini Yoga class ends with a long deep relaxation in Corpse Pose. This time allows your body to integrate and get the maximum benefit from all the effort you have made.

How to do It

LIE FLAT on your back, legs placed about twelve inches apart, feet relaxed.[8] Rest your arms loosely at your sides with the palms facing up. Close your eyes. Feel the gentle pull of gravity. Give in to it. Let your body know it doesn't have to move, or even prepare to move. You can tell your body to relax, and it will.

Here's one way to do it: Consciously, deliberately direct your body, part by part, to relax, all the way from the tip of your toes to the top of your head. Tell yourself to relax every nerve, every muscle, every cell of your body. Silently think: "Relax my feet, relax my legs, relax my thighs, relax my hips," and so on. Tell each of your organs and all your glands to relax. As the muscles relax, the breath will, too. As the breath slows and the body relaxes, let go of every feeling. Let go of the stress of life. You don't have to respond to any impulse. Neither fear nor excitement can move you. Simply float in peace and equanimity. As the Buddhists say, "There's no place to go, there's nothing to do," except relax. Become an observer of all that goes on and flows through you. Remain absolutely motionless. That is the condition. No bodily movement whatsoever.

However, be totally aware of your breath. With your eyes closed, watch it flow in and out, but don't try to control it.

"In all other postures, we imprison our breath, but in Corpse Pose it is free, relaxed. Imagine that you are not even in your body; just keep the little silver cord connecting you. Be dead. This is an opportunity to practice receiving grace."[9]

The most difficult thing to relax is the mind. Keep it perfectly still, free from all thoughts and ideas, as if you were in deep sleep. "When you can maintain this Asana, lying motionless, as if you were dead, for only fifteen minutes, free from all thoughts and activity, the body will get rid of all strain and tiredness, mental fatigue will vanish, and your mind will be fresh and energetic."[10]

Be sure to get up from Corpse Pose (or sleep or any deep meditation) slowly and gradually, taking a few long deep breaths and stretching your body in all directions.

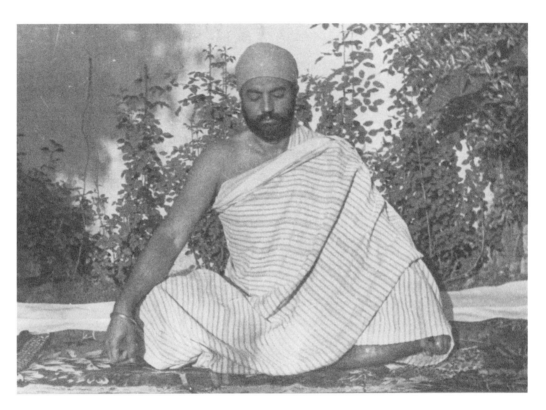

To be calm is the highest achievement of the self.

—YOGI BHAJAN

4

STRETCHING THE SPINE

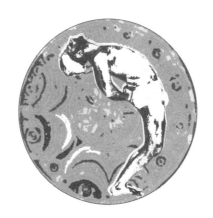

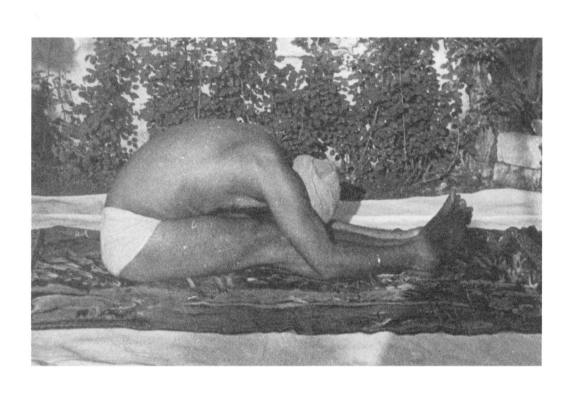

Life Nerve Stretch

Want a slender waistline? Get rid of unwanted fat round waist and belly?
Sit down and practice this asana instead of eating peanut butter and jelly.
You'll stay healthy and young with a flexible spine
Just be patient and give yourself time.
It's not just one stiff rod you're bending now
But a series of small bones that movement allow.
In addition to making the spine flexible, which is simply grand,
This stretch invigorates the muscles and nerves of legs and hands,
Fights diabetes, diarrhea, sciatica, and constipation.
Practice only once or twice a day to begin, in anticipation
Of the time you can repeat five to seven times; Ah, what jubilation!

Try it in the evening, when spine is more relaxed
But even when successful, only five to seven times, max.
Slowly exhale as forward you bend
Staying relaxed, grab your toes (if you can)
Keep legs stretched straight—don't bend your knees
Aim your forehead down, do it all with ease.
Nothing is forced, just stretch your life nerve
As your spine loosens up, it will lose that wrong curve.

Slow and steady wins the race,
Knees learning to stay in their proper place.

It's hard for everyone (except youngsters), but the benefits abound.
Keep practicing, 'til you can easily keep your knees on the ground.
If at first you can't keep your legs straight, don't despair
The results you'll get are worth all the care.

Hold with breath out five seconds or ten
Then release the toes, inhale, and sit up again.

How to do It

IF YOU can't reach your toes without bending your knees, just hold on to your ankles or legs, wherever you can. The important thing is to stretch the life nerve (sciatic nerve) that runs from the back of the heel all the way up the back of the leg. As you become more flexible, and can easily reach your toes, bend your elbows and put them on the floor outside your knees.

Remember not to force your body, rather allow it to stretch forward, a little at a time.

A raised kundalini will give you grace of motion.

Life fills every cell so you are able to move smoothly with an

awareness of the rhythm and music of all your environments.

The kundalini makes you alive and graceful,

not rigid like some kind of death.

—YOGI BHAJAN

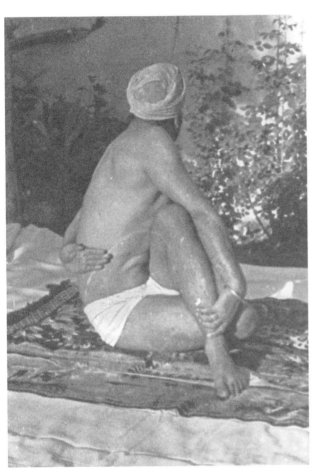

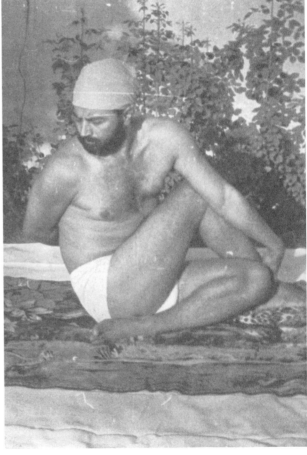

Spinal Twist

MATSYENDRASANA

Rejuvenate your spine, remove rheumatism of the back and hip
No more constipation—and indigestion you'll whip
Plus: you cure defects of liver and spleen
When you do the Twist (not so hard as it seems!)
It perfectly stimulates the nerves and muscles of both sides of the spine
Practice once a day in winter, twice in summertime
    (of course you do both left and right sides).

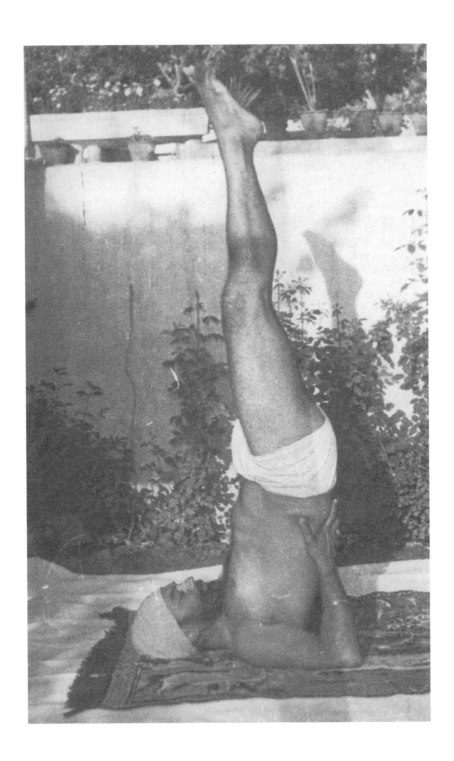

Shoulder Stand

(OR TOPSY-TURVY POSE)

BIPARIT KARANI

Rest your arteries every day,
Turn yourself upside down this easy way
Make your skin glow, build stamina and grace
Bring blood circulation to your beautiful face.

Daily practice when you are young, yogic texts advise,
Will give you lifelong youth and vigor (yes it will—if you're wise),
Keeps the body young and energetic, despite each passing year,
Resists the withering of the skin, and the graying of the hair—
    those signs of aging we all fear.

More benefits to Shoulder Stand, let me expound:
It removes constipation, indigestion, and anemia,
That's what the yogis have found.
Wait, there's even more to tell,
Shoulder Stand neutralizes toxins in the system as well.
On your back with your legs held high
Support your hips, reach your toes to the sky
You're toning up the Soma Granth (the fountainhead of
    "life energy" that resides in the head).
Ideal to do Shoulder Stand before going to bed.

Excellent for circulation, the yogis say,
Since, weakened from fighting gravity all day,
Blood vessels and arteries will thank you, for sure
When they recoup lost energy with the Shoulder Stand cure.

"Make it a shoulder stand, not a neck stand. Have your hands as low toward the ground as possible with the elbows as close together as possible so that your biceps are supporting your whole body. Otherwise, the weight of the body collapses on your neck."[1]

How to do It

LIE FLAT on your back, keeping your legs straight and arms resting at your sides. Slowly raise both legs up about thirty degrees. Then catch the hips with both hands for support and raise the lower body further up until it is perpendicular to the earth.

Note: If you cannot do Shoulder Stand as described, try this simpler form: Lie on your back close to a wall, and use the wall as a support for your legs, as you raise the lower half of your body up to the correct angle. (One text says to be sure to drink plenty of water beforehand.)

Perfect Shoulder Stand

SARBANGASANA

Glands are the guardians of your health and beauty
Taking care of them is your human duty.
You revitalize thyroid, parathyroid, tonsils,
and salivary (protective) glands
When straight like an arrow on your shoulders you stand.

How to do It

THIS IS what the texts call the "perfect" form of Shoulder Stand, and if you
can do it, it promises outstanding benefits.

The technique is slightly different from the previous Shoulder Stand in that
in this version, the legs and thighs are in line with the shoulders (rather than
in line with the waist), and the whole body is poised on the shoulders. In Perfect Shoulder Stand the hands are placed on the back for support instead of
at the hips. Another variation of this posture is what you do with your hands.
They can be kept on the ground parallel to each other or tangled together at
the wrists and pressed on the back, helping to keep the body erect on the
shoulders. Maximum time for simply holding this posture is five minutes.

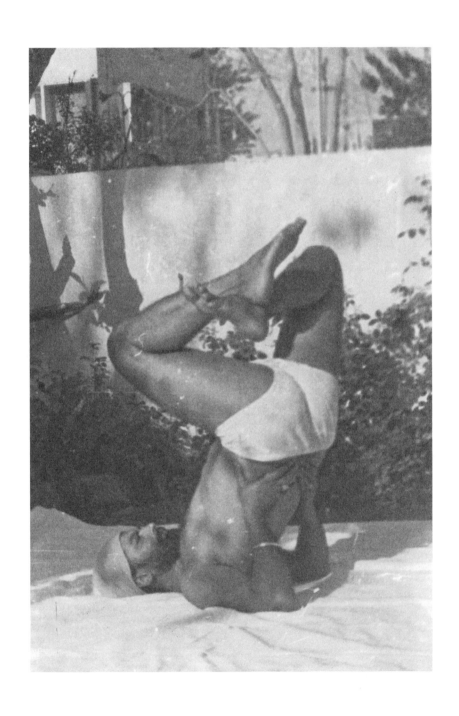

Shoulder Stand Lotus

PADMA SARVANGASAN)

Legs are placed in Lotus, after you're in Shoulder Stand—
Remember to support your lower back with your hands.
If you wish, you can start out in Lotus, before lying down flat
Then raise your body up, and that takes care of that.

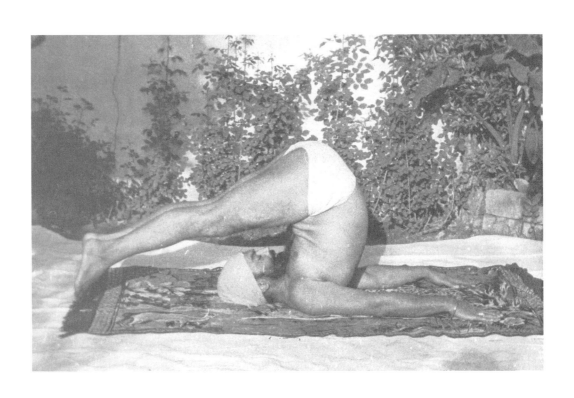

Plough

HALASANA

Get rid of surplus fat, correct your liver and spleen
Strengthen your heart—Plough keeps you young and keen.
This pose is only for teens and older,
Master it slowly and later get bolder.
From flat on your back, gradually raise the legs thirty degrees,
Pause, then continue, lift thirty more 'til it's a breeze
To slowly lower straight legs over behind your head
    resting your toes on the ground.
You inhale coming up and over, exhale slowly, very slowly,
    as you gracefully lie back down.
Three to five times both morning and night.
(Texts presume you already do Shoulder Stand right.)
Muscles of thighs, pelvic region, abdomen, and heart
Are invigorated, surplus fat will depart,
Prevent loss of appetite, diabetes, and constipation,
Good results predicted for glands in your throat
    when you practice this configuration.
(Arms can remain at your sides throughout,
Or you can bring them back behind your head.
Another variation you can think about:
Interlace your fingers to support your head instead.)

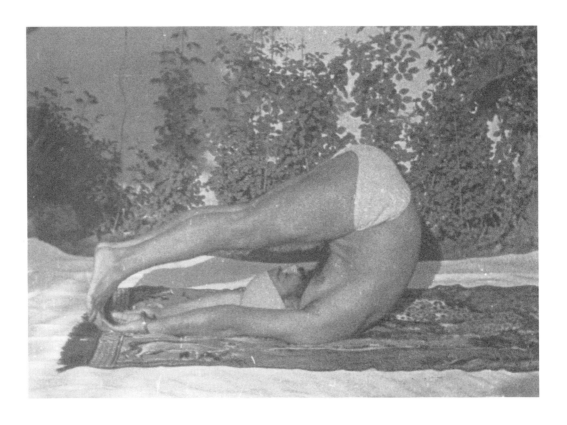

A guru, a teacher, a messiah, a master is a technical how-how man. If it

doesn't work for you, find another technique; and if that doesn't work,

find another technique. Every part doesn't fit every car.

—YOGI BHAJAN

How to do It

COME INTO Plough Pose from Shoulder Stand. Your back should be perpendicular to the ground; then lower your feet back behind your head. Most common arm position is with the hands clasped in the opposite direction from the feet.[2]

Note: In some Kundalini Yoga kriyas we walk the feet out to the sides a few inches, then back together several times while in Plough Pose, keeping the arms lying alongside the body, not toward the head.

In another kriya I remember lying prone, then inhaling into Plough, exhaling and returning to prone, then inhaling to sit up and reach for the toes (as in Life Nerve Stretch), then exhaling back down prone; continuing this sequence about twenty-six times. (Palms are facedown on the floor in the prone position, as distinct from Corpse Pose.) One source claims that Plough also adjusts the functioning of the kidneys and pancreas (as well as the liver) and regulates the thyroid, balancing the metabolism.

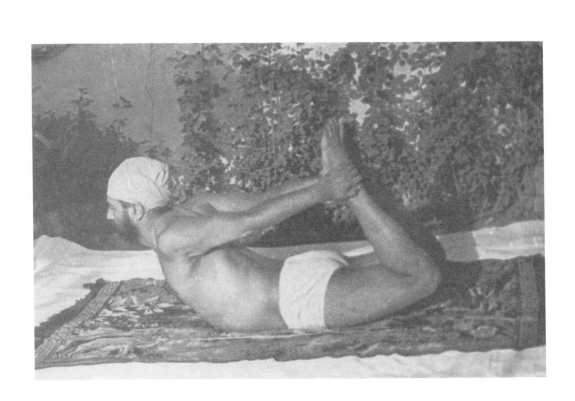

Bow

DHANURASANA

Liver, spleen, intestines, large and small,
Abdominal muscles—defects in any of these are solved
When you balance on your belly, feet together, ankles high;
To the causes of diabetes, rheumatism, and fat on the
abdomen, you can cheerfully say good-bye.

How to do It

LIE DOWN flat on your stomach. Bend your knees and push them toward your back; catch hold of your ankles with both hands, keeping the feet together. Lift up your head and chest. Ideally the body is balanced on the abdomen only, and the neck is stretched back as in Cobra. Don't put pressure on your neck or strain it.

TIPS: Your knees can come apart a little bit, but your toe joints and heels stay together. Keeping the heels together will help you to access the spine evenly so you're not compressing one area. Don't put emphasis on lifting the head—the focus is across the chest. Feel an even stretch from neck to pelvis, across the thighs.[3]

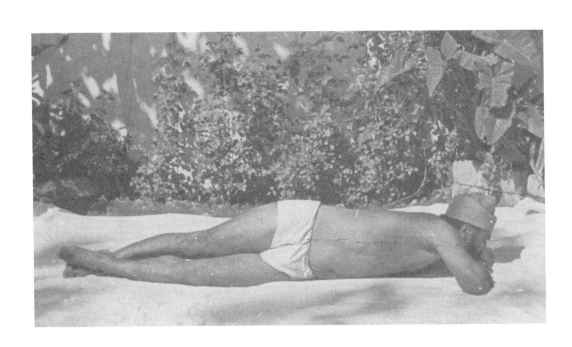

Special Twist

MOGRASANA

The description of this Special Twist has somehow eluded
But, since we have the photo, it should be included.
I would hazard a guess it's for the hips and the spine and works on circulation.
I trust that description is fine, and will not cause complications.

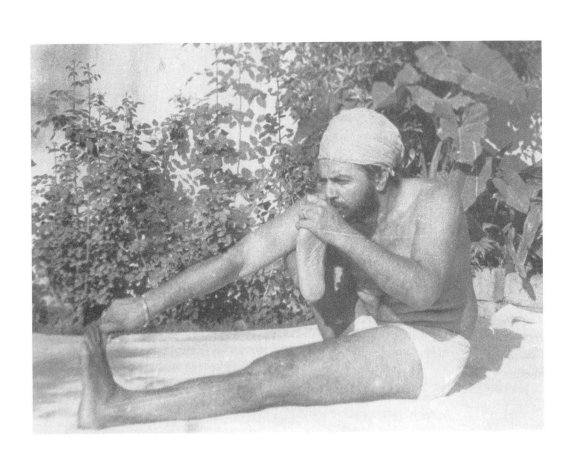

Ek Pad Dhanurasana

❧

Forgive me if I give this one a pass
Though I vaguely remember Yogi Bhajan did teach it in class.
That was in the early days, as he tested our mettle.
Myself, for just breathing and chanting I'll happily settle!
Note, however, if you are pretzel prone,
This posture is great to rid children of defects in the bones
Especially in their hands and feet.
Your liver gets stronger, appetite will increase,
Rheumatism of aging hands and feet, and even sciatica run away
When you add Ek Pad Dhanurasana to your practice each day.
One leg stretched straight, hold the toes with the opposite hand.
Bend the other leg up to your thigh, grab the toes. My, you look grand!
Pull that foot up to your ear
(Or at least, try to get near),
If not the ear, the nose will do—
Change sides and repeat, on each side, a few.

Congratulations, I'm truly impressed—
At least you tried, and did your best!

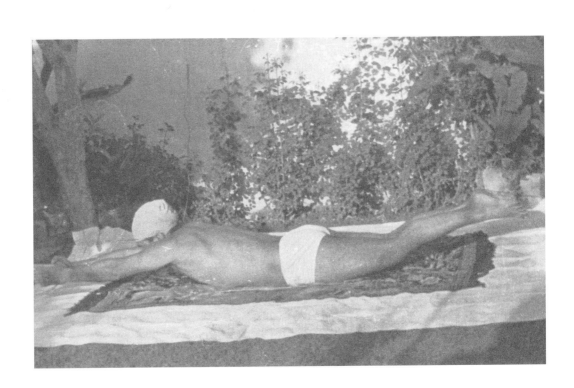

Boat

NAUKASANA

Your lungs will love you, stomach flab will flee,
Digestion improve, constipation relieved,
Body so light and agile you'll think you can float
When you lift yourself into this Boat.
Raise your arms and legs slowly, as high as you can
Increase blood circulation, whether woman or man.

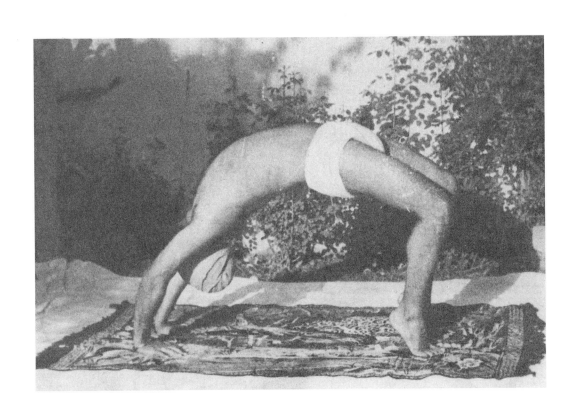

Half-Wheel

ARDHA-CHAKRASANA

❦

Half a wheel is better than none!
In fact, it's more than enough to keep you young,
Providing the benefits of both Cobra and Bow,
You are bent over backwards, with head dropped low.

With the full strength of inverted palms,
Make an effort, inch by inch, don't have any qualms.
From flat on your back raise waist, head and chest
(Of course in between, you'll want to take rest.)
"You may die, but you'll never grow old,
When you have a flexible spine," we're told.
Two to ten seconds is all you hold—
No matter how brave, no matter how bold,
Maximum, practice twice in any half-day
    (three to five times if the weather is cold).+

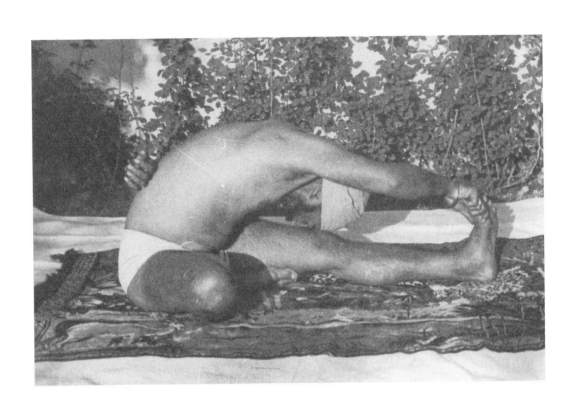

Janu–Sis Asan

❀

Want to be taller, young girls and lads?
Cure sciatica, lumbago, and piles, you mothers and dads?
Janu-Sis Asan assists with these ills it is claimed,
The list is impressive, kindly let me explain:
Removes weakness and lethargy; with appetite up, meals will last longer,
You'll feel great, as muscles 'round your navel get stronger.

How to do It

FOLD ONE leg under, with the heel in the perineum and the sole on the opposite thigh. Firmly place the other leg out straight—try not to bend your knee—and grab onto the outstretched toes. Fold the body forward, pulling down with your arms. Lead with your heart, not with your head. Keep bending until, ideally, your forehead touches down on the knee.

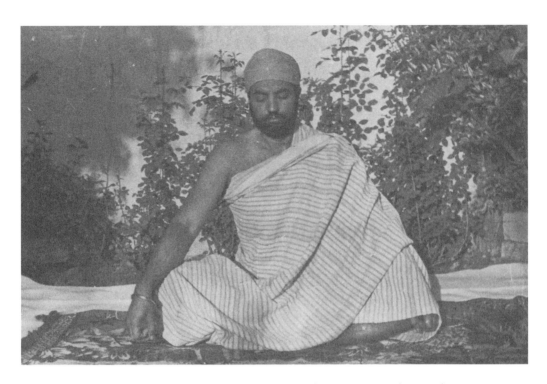

Yoga is a science of reality and experiential proof

of the sacredness of all life.

You are holy if you have nine holes and you watch what goes in and out!

If it's a conscious act, you are holy. If it's an emotional act,

you are unholy. If it's a commotional act, you are insane.

If it's an unconscious act, you are an idiot.

—YOGI BHAJAN

ANIMAL NATURE

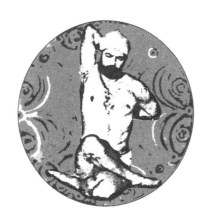

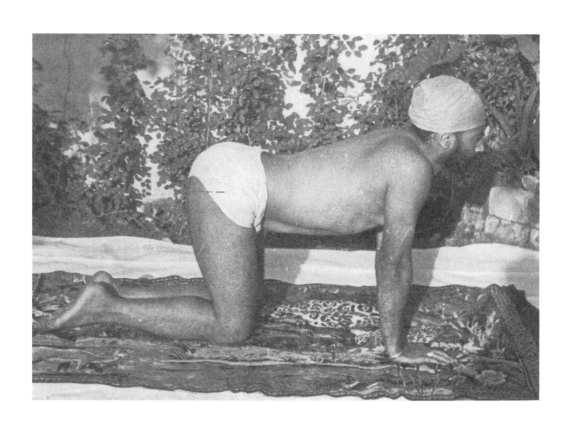

Cats and Cows

❧

In our yoga practice, cats and dogs aren't raining,
There are no serpents sunning on rocks
But we twist ourselves into cows and monkeys,
Lions and frogs—even peacocks.
It's not a menagerie, though it sounds like one
With many barnyard animals—and then some.
When the yogis gave these postures animal names, we joyfully assume,
They were cleverly trying to make our human consciousness bloom.

Putting cats and cows together might not happen on a farm,
But when we alternate these two yogic postures, it doesn't do any harm.
In fact with the rapid, fluid motion of the spine
(In Cat your head goes down, while your back arches high
Combined with the Cow who looks to the blue
With buttocks up and spine slumped in a U),
You stimulate the reservoir of energy called kundalini
That's eagerly waiting to be released (and only rhymes with linguini)!

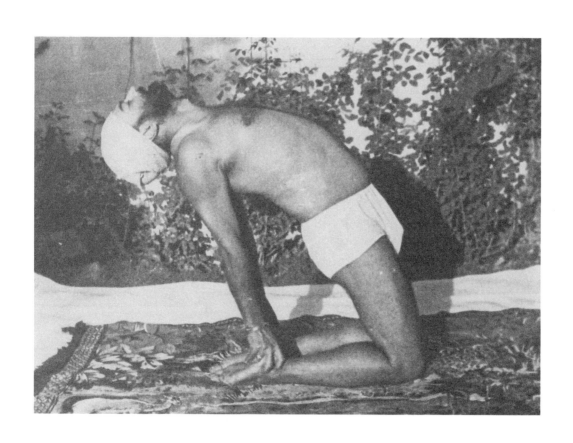

Camel

USTRASANA

Make your spine flexible, muscles and nerves grow strong
Increase your sexual control so you won't go wrong
Ten to fifteen seconds with breath held out,
That's what Camel is all about.
Inhale, relax, rest, and repeat twice or thrice—
Do it faithfully, do it nice:
You'll remain youthful and never feel old
If this Camel Posture you hold.

How to do It

KNEELING, FEEL that your knees are anchored into the ground. Leave your
head up while you bend backward. Your head will be the last thing to bend
back. Reach back and grasp your heels, keeping the hands and arms straight
as pillars. Emphasize lifting your chest. Keep your shoulders down, and your
thighs pressed forward. Exhale as you are bending backward; hold the breath
out ten to fifteen seconds then inhale as you come out of the position. Rest,
and repeat two or three times.

   (When Camel is done as a part of a kriya [a combined set of actions], you
may be doing Breath of Fire or Long Deep Breathing while holding the position for one or two minutes.)

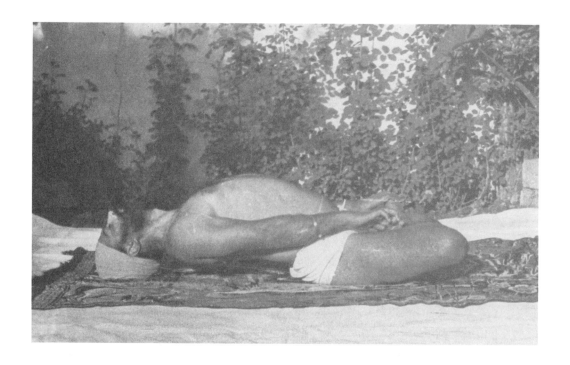

WARNING

If you have a bad neck, avoid Fish Pose—it puts too much strain on the neck.

Fish

MATSYA MUDRA OR MATSYASANA

Fish don't have shoulders, so these two asanas go hand in hand:
To absorb all the calcium your body needs,
     do both Fish Pose and Shoulder Stand.
The way this works is a glandular thing,
Balanced secretion of the four parathyroids—these two asanas bring.

From Lotus Pose (if you can) lie flat down on your back
     keeping your knees down
Arch your back way up so the very top center of your head
     rests on the ground
Your knees and your head carry the weight
As you hold on to the toes of opposite feet.

Hold for only thirty seconds when you first become a Fish
You can gradually increase the time,
     three to five minutes (but no more), if you wish.
No matter how much milk you drink, or oranges, nuts, and onions you eat,
If the parathyroids aren't working right,
     even calcium injections won't succeed.
For digestive problems, and a whole list of other ills
When glands undersecrete, doctors may advise you, "Take pills."
On the other hand, when the parathyroid excessively secretes,
High blood pressure is caused and so I repeat:
Glands are the guardians of your health and beauty,
Take good care of them, it is your duty.

TIP: Emphasize lifting your chest off the ground and letting your arms pull,
     so that you help ease the full weight on the head and neck.

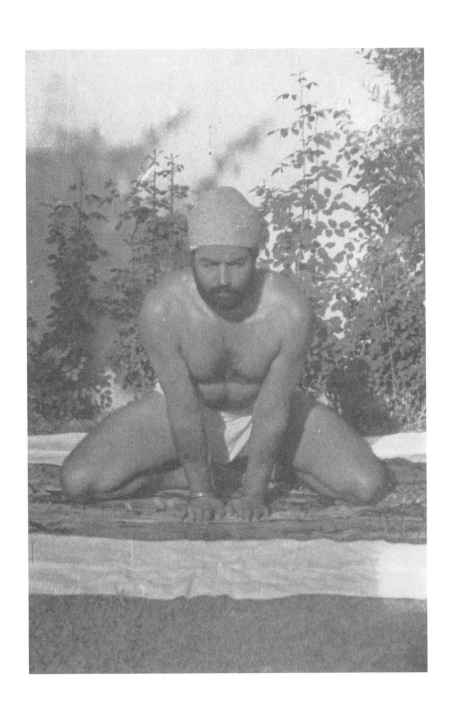

Frog

MANDAKASANA

Protruding belly? Short of breath? Want to jump and hop?
Frog Pose unifies prana and apana,[1]
   slowly build up to twenty-six repetitions, then stop!
Squatting keeping heels "glued" together, rise up and down on the toes
(The variation we usually practice looks different
   from what the picture shows.)

Inhale, straighten your legs as your hips go up and your head goes down,
Fingertips, placed between the knees, stay firmly on the ground.
Alternate from squatting to straight as Frog Pose you apply,
Transforming and elevating sex energy from lower chakras to high.[2]
Whether you do them slow, or do them fast
Frogs solve stomach ailments, and eliminate gas.

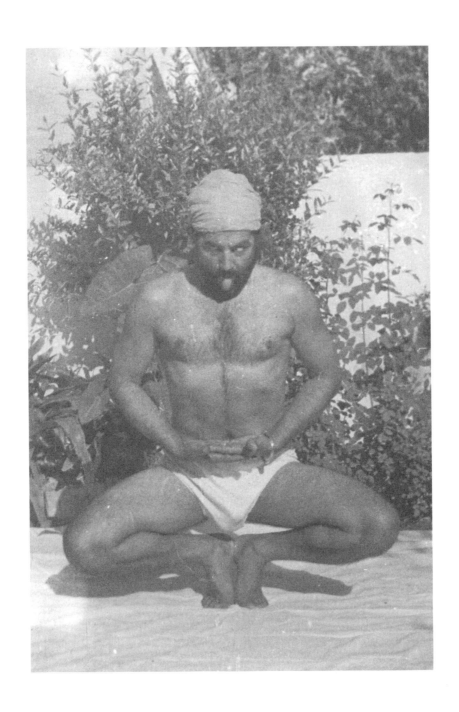

Lion
SIHNASANA

The kingly lion strikes terror in the hearts of his foes
No wonder they fear, if a lion strikes this awful pose!
If you can't crouch on toes with feet and heels together as prescribed
At least pull your chin in, gaze at the third eye,
   and open your mouth really wide—
Stick your tongue way, way out, hands can go on your knees or lap
Ideally: feet straight and raised with heels touching the anus,
   yet both heels stay in contact.
Have a sore throat? Problem with teeth, tongue, or jaws?
Use Lion Pose to become fearless, and eliminate these flaws.
In addition, develop virility and power, even make your voice clear.
A unique feature of Lion, all three locks engage automatically here.
If you are timid and want to improve your eyesight, too,
Emulate the king of the jungle and see what the Lion can do for you.

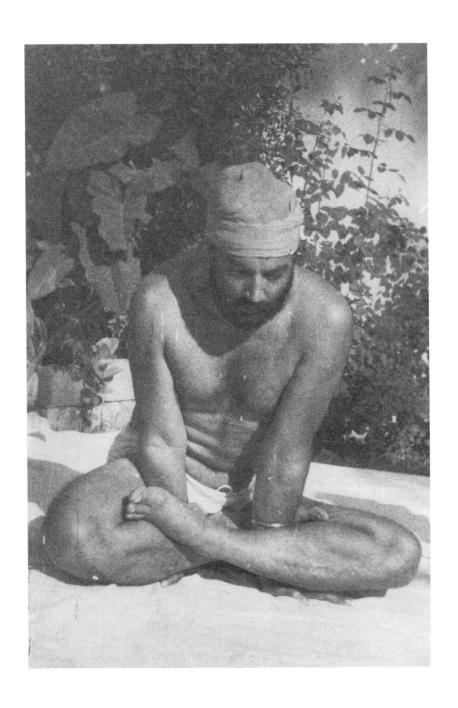

Cock

KUKKUTASANA

Feeling lethargic, wimpy and bland?
This pose will revitalize the nerves of your wrists and your hands
Chest and shoulders are helped out too
When this asana is regularly practiced by you.

If for some reason you feel inclined
To attempt this posture, keep in mind
You start with your right leg on your left thigh
And the left leg goes on the right.
Insert both hands through the bend of your knees,
Using only fingers and palms, raise your body up with ease.
Well, perhaps it's not easy, but try anyway.
Hold yourself steady and attempt to stay
One to three minutes, then rest and repeat.
For people of all professions and trades, this can't be beat,
 Especially if to writer's cramp you're prone
 Or you use your arms a lot on the job or at home.

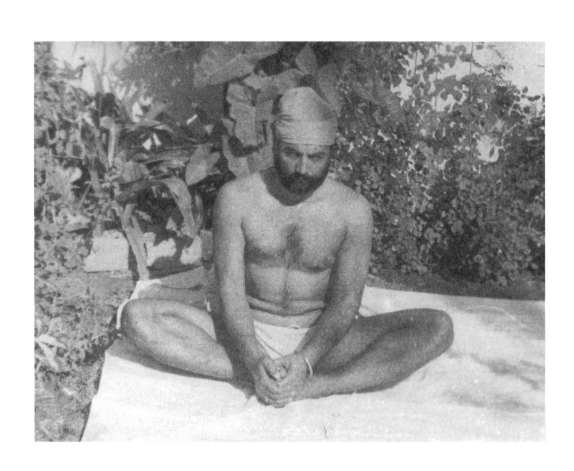

Butterfly

GORABHASANA (GORAKSASANA) OR BHADRASANA

To expand and strengthen the nerves of the knees and the pelvic region,
This Butterfly loves to fly in any season
Soles of the feet pressed together, held firmly by hands,
Helps maintain celibacy, or retentive power if you're a man.
Ideal exercise for pregnant women to do
So childbirth is eased when the time comes for you.
In Kundalini Yoga, we let the Butterfly rise,
Happily fluttering the knees—good for both girls and guys.
Keep the backbone erect, do your best
Close to your body, feet are pressed.

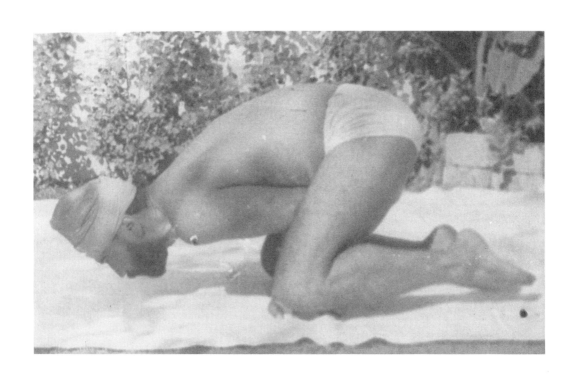

Peacock

MAYURASANA

❧

Your digestion will be the best, your stomach will be your friend,
Intestines and kidneys will never trouble you, digestive problems will end.
In perfected Peacock Posture, the body does not bend.
Eyesight defective? Want to benefit your lungs?
Glowing praises of the virtues of Peacock have been sung.
Peacock's power can enable you to digest virtually anything on your diet.
'Tis said peacocks can even eat poison (we do not recommend you try it!).

How to do It

"SIT ON your heels (or your toes). Place the palms away from the knees, keeping the wrists close to each other; the palms will remain inverted with fingers toward the knees. Next rest the body on the hands, keeping the elbows on the region of the navel. Now try to raise the lower half of the body as far above ground-level as possible, the head and legs remaining straight. With gradual success, the feet will rise about eight inches above the point of the navel—thus showing the body like a peacock. With practice (only three or four attempts at a time—holding only four or five seconds) you can hold for a maximum of ten seconds."[3] (The book says, "without breath.") Use the power of your arms, shoulders, and navel to lock yourself straight, parallel to the ground.[4]

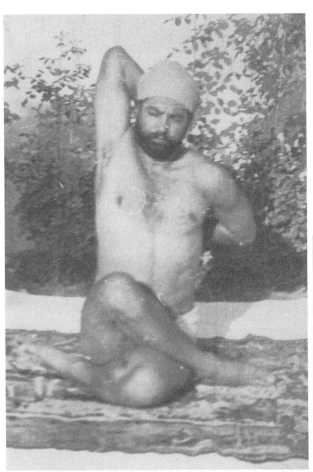

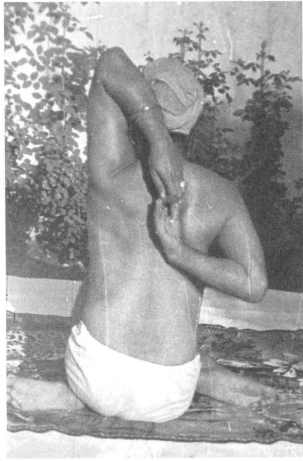

Cow-Face

GOMUKHASANA

Why it's called Cow-Face, I haven't a clue
But it strengthens the spine and does other things too:
For those who are brahmacharya (celibate and contained)
This posture helps ensure vows are maintained.
Amorous or exciting thoughts that might overpower the mind
Are repelled by grasping your hands this way from behind.
Amazingly, about Gomukhasana, the yogis also say this:
"It helps in the cure of insomnia, sciatica, piles,
rheumatism of the leg and urethritis!"

How to do It

CROSS YOUR right leg over the left, so that the right thigh rests on the left, and your right heel is beside the left buttock. Your left heel should press upon the right buttock. The right knee is over the left knee. Reach behind you with your left hand bent behind your back, palm facing out. Bend your right arm so that your right elbow points to the sky and your right hand, palm facing your back, grasps (ideally) your left hand. Even if the hands can't reach all the way, keep gently reaching! Try to keep your head from tilting forward. After holding the position for a few seconds, you can reverse it by changing arms and legs.

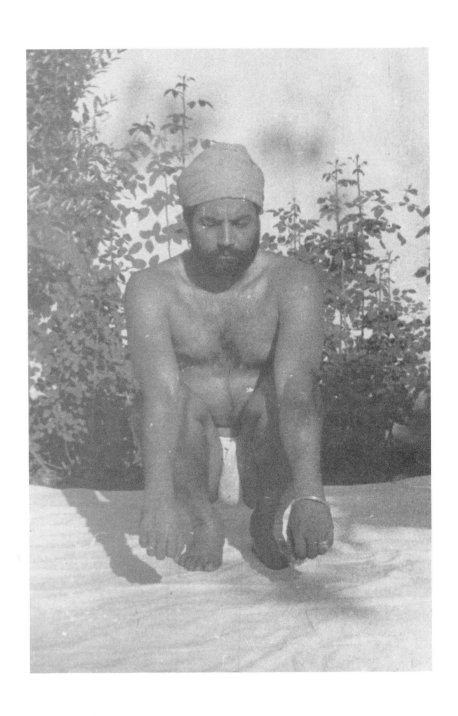

Crow

KAKASANA

Much more than the simple squat that you see,
Crow improves circulation in thighs, buttocks, calves, neck, and knees.
When you sit this way, you take up less space,
It's useful if you find yourself in a crowded place.
During the six procedures of yogic cleansing, Crow is employed.
It gives flexibility and agility, so other asanas you can fully enjoy.

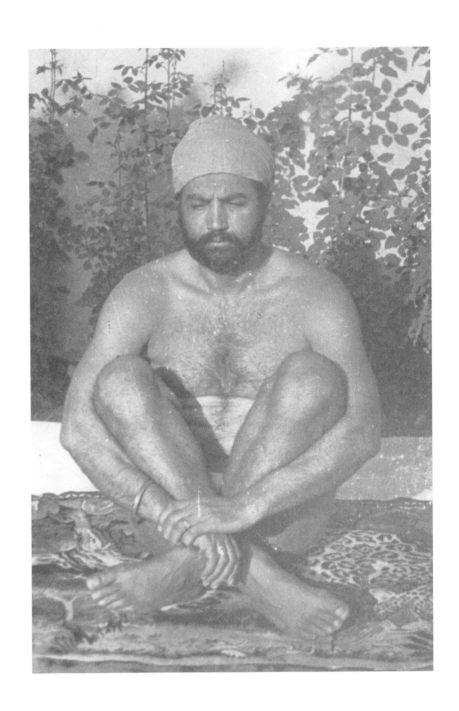

Monkey Meditation

We all strive to calm the monkey mind:
What you do with your body has an effect in kind.
Eyes closed in contemplation
Avoiding any desire or temptation,
As thoughts come in, let them go by—
This is a meditation anyone can try.
Let the breath be smooth, long and deep
Your mind becomes calm, the slower you breathe—
Think SAT as you inhale; exhale think NAM;
Guaranteed tranquility for any Harry, Sally, or Tom.

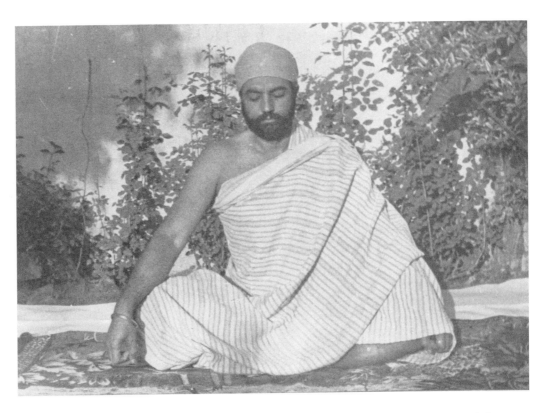

Creative Meditation is that every moment you exist as a part of the

universe, the whole universe becomes a part of you.

—YOGI BHAJAN

6

ALL BENT INTO SHAPE

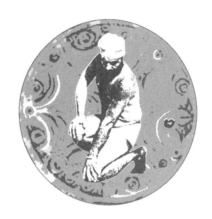

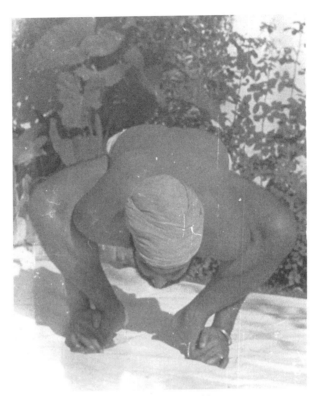

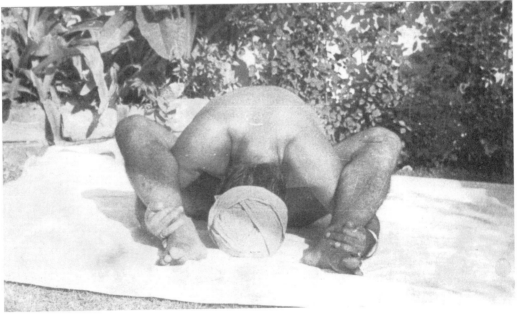

Chair

KACHUVASANA

Some chairs are comfortable; some are not.
Here's an exercise to test what you've got!
Just keep trying, until you succeed
With firm determination, here's how to proceed:
Stand up, then bend your knees, feet apart flat on the ground
Reach down in front between your thighs, wrap your arms back and around
Hands on top of your feet, head up—there's more,
Keep your back flat, parallel to the floor.

Hold two or three minutes with Breath of Fire
If to energize yourself you aspire.

(If you're very flexible and adventure bound
Bend all the way over, hands on your ankles
Forehead on the ground.)

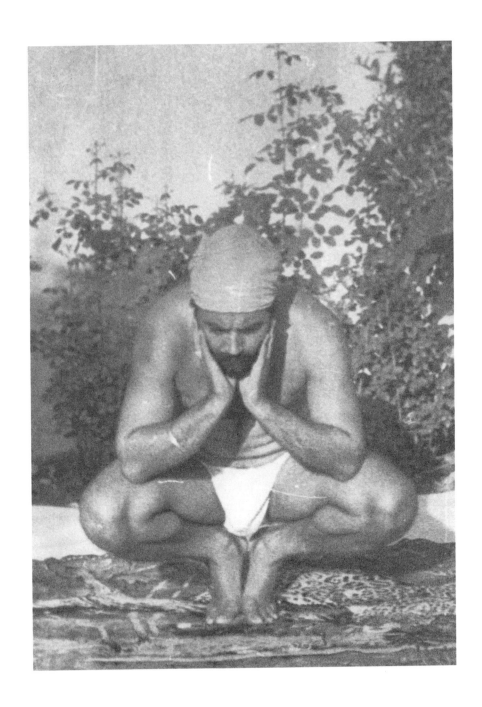

On His Toes
PROSCHITASANA

As a teacher he keeps us on our toes,
Perhaps it started when he learned this pose.
Not "The Thinker" immortalized in stone—
But an independent planner with a mind of his own
Charting the future to benefit mankind—
Wise men seek his counsel when they're in a bind.

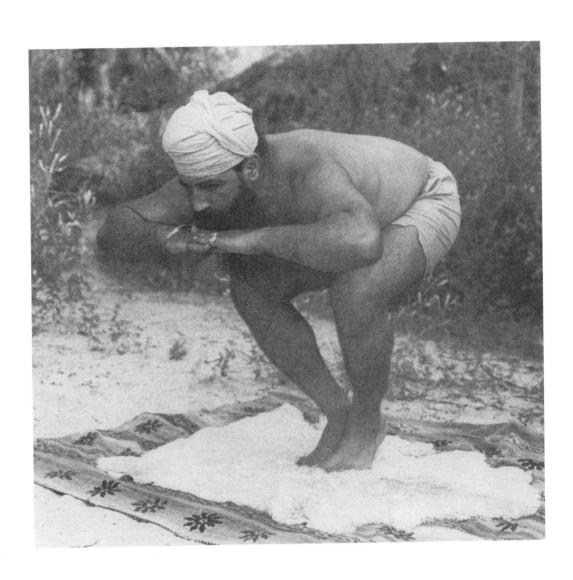

Squatting Posture
UTTKUTASANA (UTKATASANA)

Of great importance in yogic science,
This posture assures celibacy compliance;
Induces semen to travel upwards, not blocked,
Brings automatic application of diaphragm lock
"Uddiyan Bandh"—relieves stomach complaints,
Relieves painful afflictions in feet and finger joints;
Essential for yogic cleansing by water and air;
It also refreshes the brain as you're squatting there.

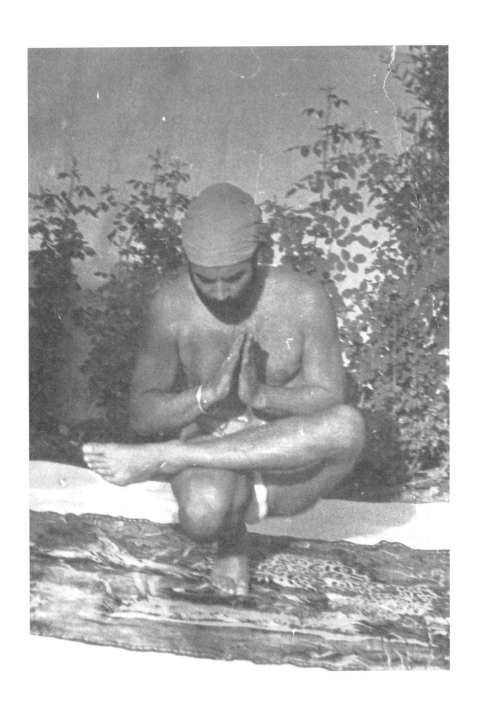

Big Toe
PADANGUSHTHASANA

You put all your weight on your toes
When, under direct supervision, you learn this pose.
Don't try it on your own, it needs a guide,
Someone to coach you right by your side.
Its benefits are clear, brahmacharya, the aim:
Developing self-control and virility all the same.
Stability of body and concentration of the mind—
Serious yogis in this posture find.

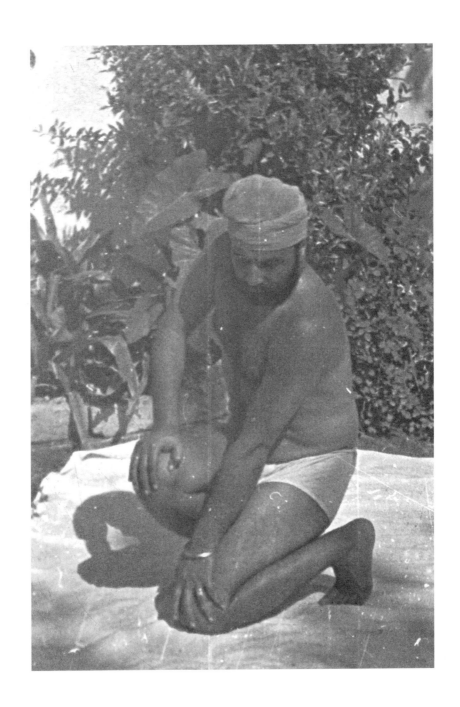

Kaga Sankha Kiryasana

(OR UDARA KARSANASANA)
BELLY-SUCTION POSTURE

This one may look simple, but don't be deceived,
Pressing each knee down toward the other foot is not easy to achieve.
You might start by squatting in Crow
(Itself beneficial for digestion, you already know).
This posture guarantees to make constipation go,
Take away lower leg pain and make your feet really strong.
Especially useful for those who trek distances long.

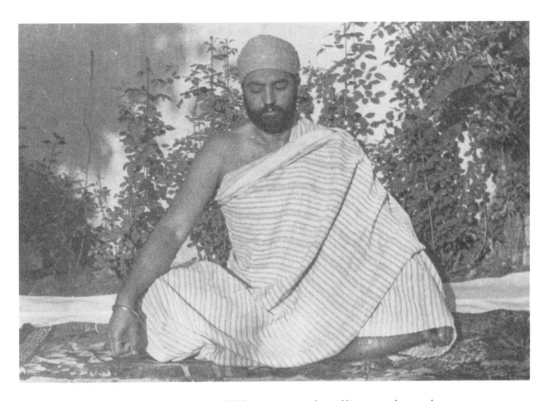

There are millions of libraries and millions of teachers,

and I have listened to them and to myself.

What I taught is nothing but rebellion against tradition

because I feel man is born in God's image, and there is nothing less to it.

—YOGI BHAJAN

7

STANDING UP RIGHT!

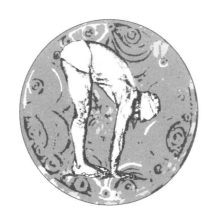

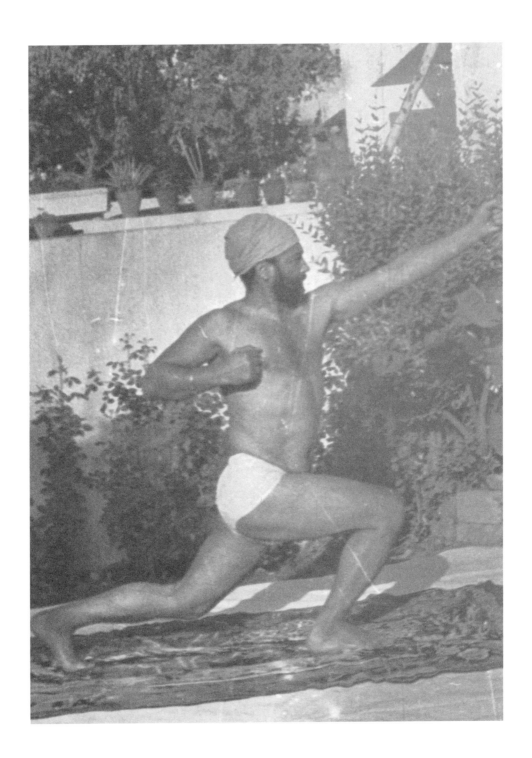

Archer

Chivalry and fearlessness, inherent in this noble warrior stance,
Physical stamina and strength in feet, thighs and arms enhanced.
Archer also puts pressure on the thigh bone,
Balancing calcium, magnesium, potassium, and sodium.

REASON

On the physical plane, we have lots of reasons for doing Archer Pose. It helps develop strength in the quadriceps and the intestines. The legs and knees are being strengthened. Outstanding physical stamina and strength are gained, while, remarkably, at the same time, there is an inner posture of feelings taking place that is equal in power to the pure physical connection of feet to the ground.

Sometimes called the Hero Posture, Archer Pose develops courage. That is its special inner gift. Plus, it is said that the need for excessive sleep disappears!

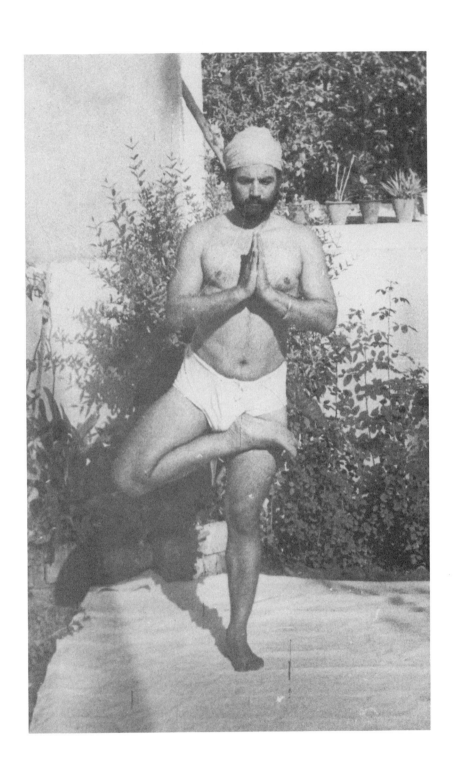

Tree
VARISHASANA

"I think that I shall never see
a poem lovely as a tree."[1]

There's balance, there's grace—
Everything in its proper place.
Concentration is required
So that you don't get tired.
Standing on one foot makes legs and ankles strong.
Remember to breathe—prana you need,
And keep both hips level where they belong.

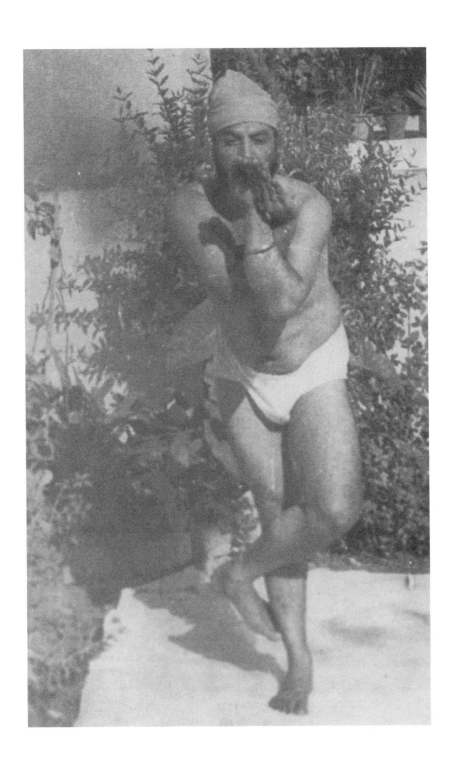

Eagle

GARUDASANA

After a long journey on foot, with Eagle relieve fatigue.
Arthritic aches and pains in joints, knees, and feet
Also disappear from elbows, arms, forearms or shoulders
When alternate sides of Garudasana you complete.
Right leg wraps around the left, arms intertwine forming the beak.
Do the Eagle, men, if from enlargement of testicles you seek relief.

TIP: For best results, lean slightly forward.

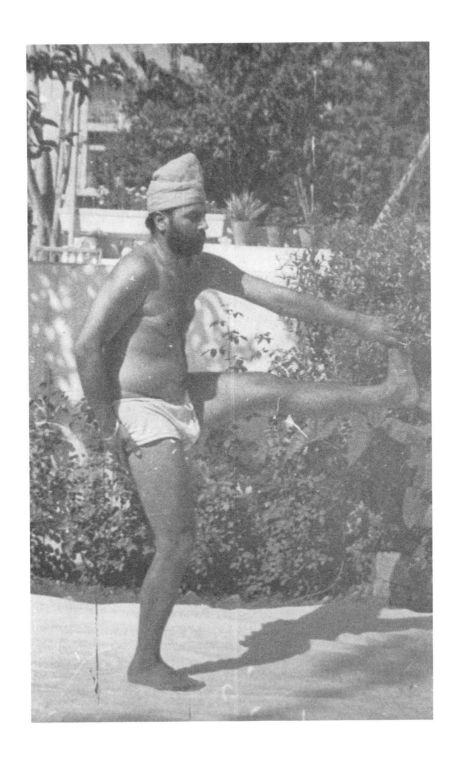

Hand-Toe

HAST PADUNGUSTHASANA

It's not the Hokey-Pokey, but first stretch one leg out straight
   as high as you can,
Catch hold of the toes, hold for a while,
   then switch sides, that's the plan.
Want to straighten your body, get taller,
   or be able to stand long hours on end?
Then practicing this Hand-Toe Posture—
   Hast Padungusthasana—is for you, my friend.

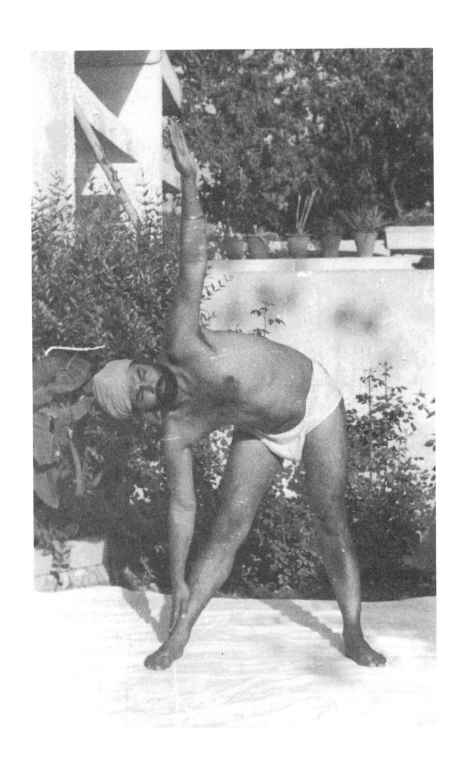

Triangle
TRIKONASANA

Again and again we find
Youth and health come from a flexible spine.
Stretching and reaching bring increased circulation,
Toning up nerves and muscles with sincere participation.

Feet comfortably, approximately three feet apart,
Stand straight in this posture, then lean over sideways to start.
Left hand reaches down toward your left toes,
Right arm reaches high in the sky, beyond your nose.
Head turns to observe fingertips up in the air,
How lovely it is to observe them there.
Both arms in a straight line, what a beautiful sight.
Gaze at your fingertips, then straighten up right.
A few times each side, alternate arms.
Up to ten to twenty repetitions, experience the charm:
Some people call this Triangle the Happy Pose;
Let joy fill your body, radiate from your soul.

How to do It

BE SURE to bend over sideways, not forward, even if you can't reach as far.
As you reach for your ankles, or the top of your foot, the important thing to
remember is that you are making a real triangle of your body. Keep your
shoulders pressed back in alignment with your back and head, so you don't
block the flow of energy.

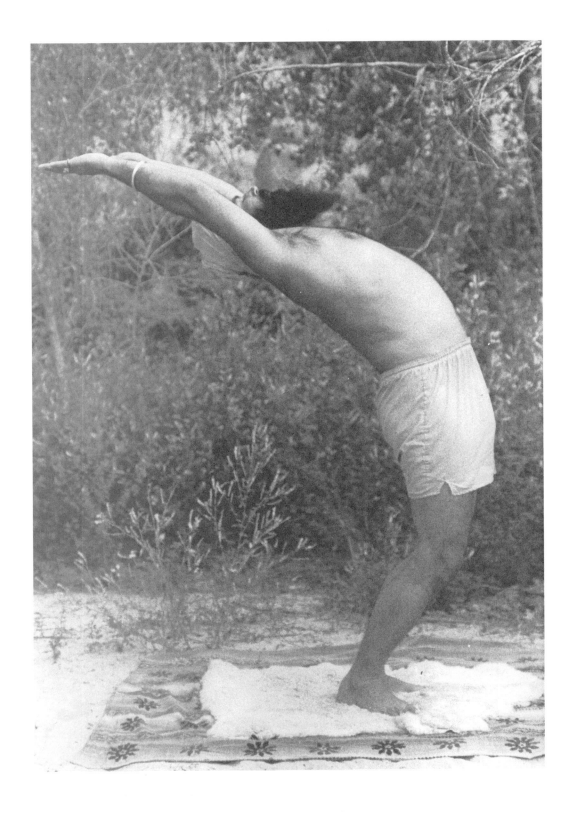

Backward Bend

URDHMAYUR DANDASANA

He has always bent over backwards to help his students grow.
Where he gets his patience and endurance, I think you should know:
He never forgets that God is the doer, he simply does God's will
With no attachment or expectation, seeing neither good nor ill—
"Unaffected by the pair of opposites," thus is a true yogi defined.
To take credit for his amazing achievements, he has always declined.

"'Someday, the day shall come, when all the Glory shall be Thine'
People will say, 'It is yours.' I shall deny, 'Not mine.'"[2]

God gave him a vision, Guru gave him a mission;
His commitment has never waned.
He gave us sacred Kundalini Yoga
And the blessing of chanting God's name.

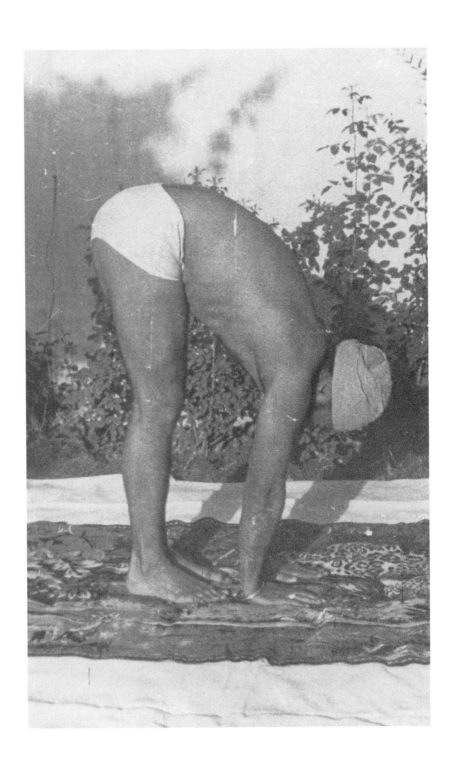

Forward Bend

HAST PAD

Illustrated here is simply Hast Pad
(Forward bend with palms on the ground);
Add some side and back stretches,
And the complete Pada-Hastasana you've found.

If your heart is strong, and your blood pressure norm,
You're encouraged to daily these stretches perform.
Want your spine straight, flexible and young, while you lose excess fat?
Get rid of constipation, anemia, indigestion and sciatica?
    Pada-Hastasana, a Whole Body Stretch, does all that.

This four-part exercise helps children grow tall,
Works on your kidneys—and that's not all
"Tones up your circulation from top to toe"
(Direct quote from the yogic text told me so!)

Stand with your heels together but toes apart
A graceful ballet routine you're about to start.

Note: When doing just the Forward Bend by itself, keep your pelvis tucked under. You may want to spread your arms wide when straightening up, to keep the chest in the lead.[3]

Whole Body Stretch

How to do It

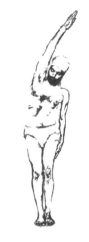

1. **Side Bend:** With both arms straight at your sides, inhale and slowly lift your left arm up over your head, keeping it straight, until you can press the elbow on the left side of the head. Then, while slowly exhaling, bend the trunk of the body to the right side, keeping the shoulder and the left hand as it is. (Straight arm touching the head. Note that the knees or legs do not bend or loosen.) Your right hand will slide toward the right heel after continued practice. Hold this position for a few seconds, keeping the breath held out, then slowly inhale and return to the standing position. Then exhale as you slowly lower the left hand down to the starting position at your side.

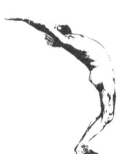

2. Repeat on the opposite side.

3. **Backward Bend:** Raise both hands slowly straight over your head while inhaling. Fix the elbows on both sides of the head and exhale slowly as you bend the trunk backward, as far as is comfortably possible. Hold this position for a few seconds with the breath out, then slowly return to the straight position as you inhale.

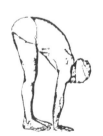

4. **Forward Bend:** Exhale and bend the trunk forward, aiming to allow your hands to touch the toes of both feet. (Eventually after practice, your head will touch your knees.) Keep your elbows next to your head as you bend. Lead with your chest, not your head, when you bend forward. Hold with the breath out, then inhale as you slowly return to the straight position. Exhale as you lower both hands down to your sides.

5. RELAX.

The physical body is a temple. Take care of it.

The mind is energy. Regulate it.

The soul is the projection. Represent it.

All knowledge is false if the soul is not experienced in the body.

—Yogi Bhajan

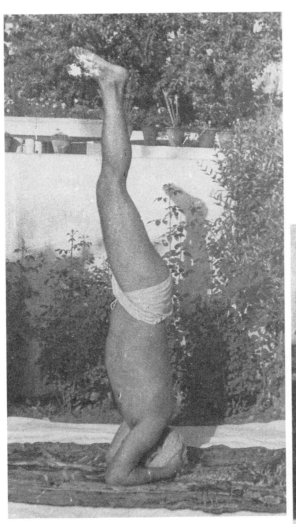

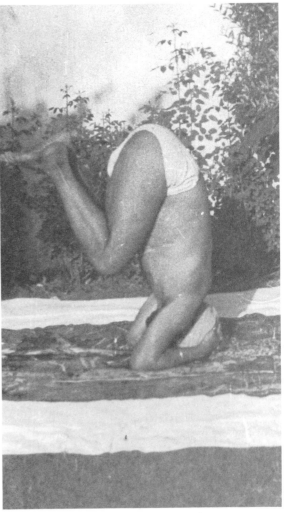

Headstand

MASTAK MUDRA OR SHIRSHANASANA
(URDH SIRSHASANA)

If you're inclined to sexual excess,
You must avoid the headstand—for your happiness.
But if you're contained, content, and controlled
Its marvelous virtues must be extolled:
Your glands, the nerves and cells of the brain
Rejoice as perfect bodily health you gain.

However, that being said,
Only under the direct supervision
Of a qualified teacher,
Should you attempt to stand on your head.

Otherwise, don't do it. Too much can go wrong
Whether you're weak or whether you're strong.
For advanced students only, and not even then
Unless you have a teacher to tell you how and when.

You can safely substitute Shoulder Stand or Plow
To get blood circulation in your head (or you can just bow).

How to do It

HEADSTAND MUST be done with a qualified teacher's supervision, because there are so many details that must be monitored to achieve proper safe alignment, and help is needed for getting in and out of the position.

When done correctly, your weight is actually more on your forearms than on your head. Fingers are laced behind your head to create a stable triangular platform. The trick in Headstand is to have the majority of the weight on the forearms.[4]

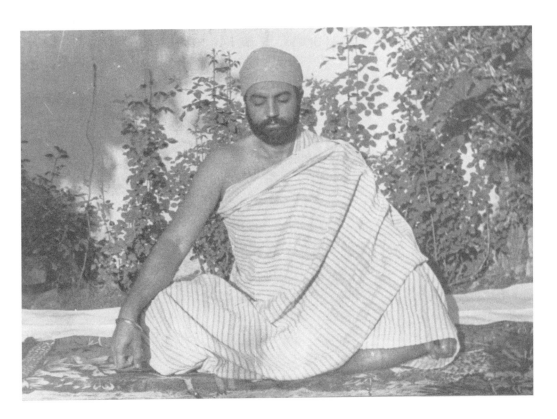

What is meditation?

When you empty yourself and let the universe come in you.

—Yogi Bhajan

8

MEDITATION POSTURES

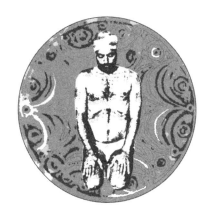

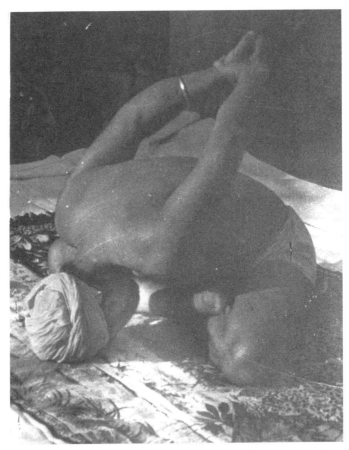

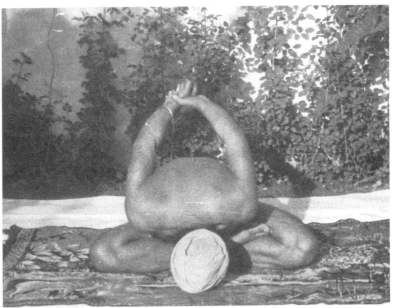

Yoga Mudra

❀

As preparation for meditation, Yoga Mudra is done.
  But that benefit is not the only one.
It works on enlarged liver or spleen,
Plus improvement in general health can be seen.

Sit on your heels, Easy Pose, or Lotus—
Yoga Mudra will help you to focus.
One hand behind your back holds the other wrist
Exhale, bend forward, let your forehead give the ground a kiss.
Arms are held high, reach for the sky,
Hold a few seconds then inhale, sit up and repeat.
As preparation for meditation Yoga Mudra can't be beat.

How to do It

WOMEN GRASP the left wrist with the right hand, men grasp the right wrist
with the left. A variation is to have the hands in Venus Lock (see glossary).
Make sure your forehead is on the ground, not the top of your head.

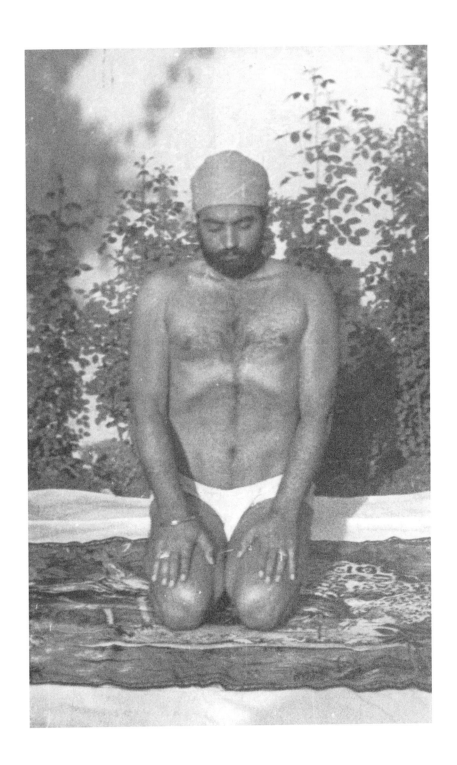

Rock Pose

(OR ADAMANT POSE)
VAJRASANA

If, from childhood, sitting on your heels,
You comb your hair every single day,
Texts advise, "No matter how old you turn,
Your hair will never turn gray."
For five minutes after each meal, breathe through your nostril right—
Even if rocks you eat, you can digest them well, morning, noon, or night.
If long hours you must keep,
Practice Vajrasan so you can get by on less sleep.
Be adamant (!) strengthen toes, legs, knees, and thighs
With heels directly underneath buttocks, or slightly off to the sides.

REASON

Muslims use Vajrasana for prayer, and the Japanese Buddhists sit in this pose for meditation. Rock Pose strengthens the pelvic muscles, which helps prevent hernia and is helpful to women in childbirth.

How to do It

IN ORDER to easily engage the Neck Lock (pulling the chin in, as in the photo), as well as other locks, try to have your pelvis balancing a straight, aligned spine.[1] One book suggests lowering the buttocks onto the insides of the feet, keeping the big toes crossed underneath.

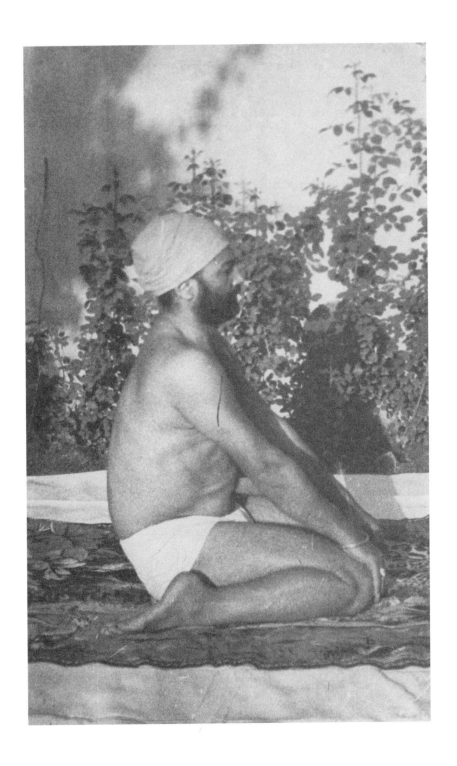

Celibate Pose

BRAHMACHARYASANA

Sit between your heels, with your bottom on the ground.
Do this before going to bed, and
    simple as it seems,
Celibate Pose will help you avoid
    debilitating wet-dreams.
It enhances virility, improves concentration, and
Calms down the libido.
It's good to practice right after meals
(Though not in a restaurant, or they'll think you're a weirdo).

    Inhaling SAT, and exhaling NAM,
    Your back gets more flexible,
    While you become calm.

    The mind follows the breath,
    And the body follows the mind
    The secret of control
    In pranayam and meditation we find.

Note: In some Kundalini Yoga kriyas, spine flexes are done in Celibate Pose. This photo shows the exhale position.

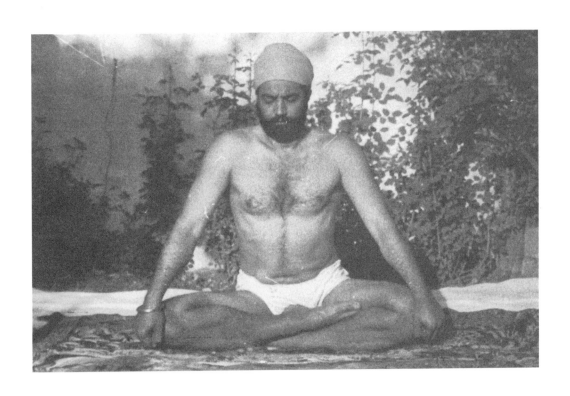

Perfect Posture

SIDDHASANA

For meditation, worship, and prayer, sitting in this posture for hours,
Yogis have attained Self-realization, and even supernatural powers.
They practice pranayam in this Perfect Pose, best results to obtain
Complete absorption, oneness with the One, Samadhi, in Siddhasan,
    is the highest aim.
Two mudras approved for the hands in this pose:
Hands in the lap—you become light and buoyant—as if the body rose.
But you get heavier with hands on the knees in Gyan Mudra
    (as the photo shows)
If you're a full-time yogi, you can go the three-hour forty-eight-minute limit,
But if you're a householder, observe moderation regarding the time you're in it.

"Mastery of this posture is attained when the yogi maintains the pose continuously for three hours and forty-eight minutes." . . . "The yogi who performs Siddhasan for twelve years, while meditating on his self and partaking of a restricted diet, attains a state of consummate perfection."[2]

How to do It

ONE SOURCE says Siddhasan is only to be practiced by men. This is probably because it requires putting the heel of the left foot against the anus, and the right heel against the testicles. Toes go between the calves and the thighs. Another description says to fold the right leg and place the sole of the right foot flat against the left thigh, with the right heel pressing the perineum (the area between the genitals and the anus). Then you fold the left leg and place the left foot on top of the right calf. Press the pelvic bone with the left heel directly above the genitals.

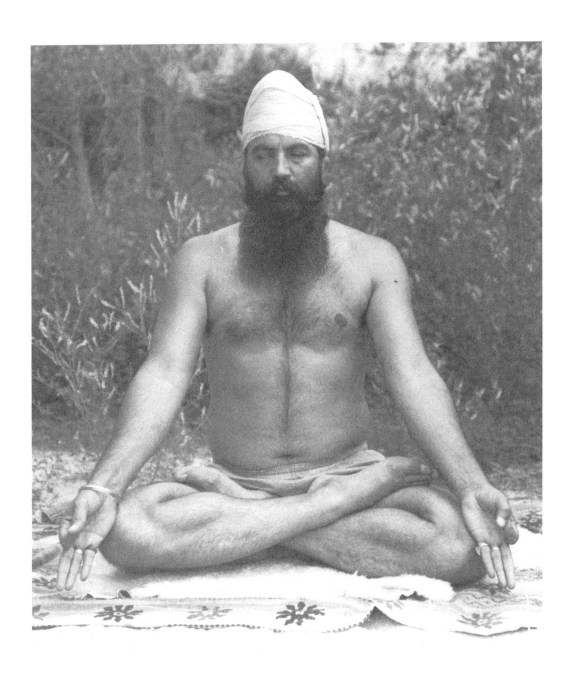

Lotus

MUKTA PADMASANA

Classic and graceful, the ultimate meditation pose
Removes defects of the legs and rheumatism woes,
Corrects curvature of the spine; it's generally sublime.
Yogic texts insist we all can master it in time.
(Practice at first with one leg still on the floor,
Hold and then switch to the other when sore.)
Eventually your legs will obey your direction
So you can do Lotus, posture of perfection.

At the root of the front teeth, put your tongue
Apply the Neck Lock, now you've begun.
When you can sit for fifteen minutes in Lotus Pose
Steadily gazing at the tip of your nose,
You're ready for the highest meditations,
You're in the best position for inner contemplation.

How to do It

TO AVOID putting too much pressure on the knee joint, always place yourself into this posture by lifting up the leg from the ankle and the knee simultaneously. Most traditions instruct starting with the right foot on the bottom.[3]

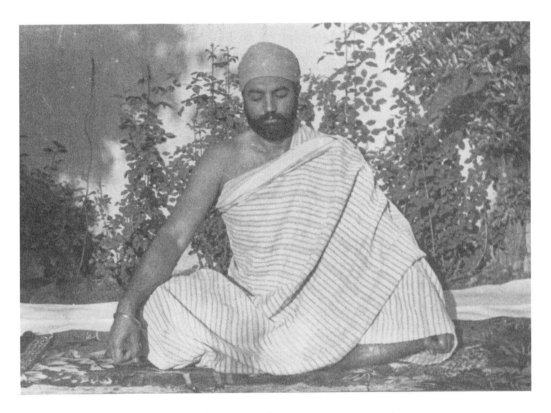

Patience gives you the power to practice;

practice gives you power that leads you to perfection.

—Yogi Bhajan

KUNDALINI YOGA KRIYAS

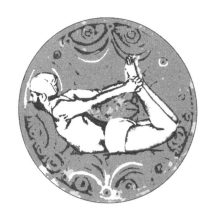

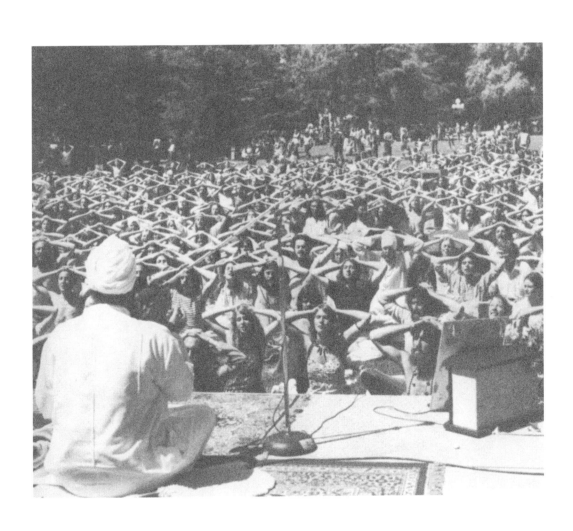

What Is a Kriya?

❧

FROM THE SANSCRIT verb *kri* (to make or to do), a kriya is a completed action. Sometimes a kriya is just one exercise, and sometimes it is a series of exercises.

A Kriya combines:

- ❧ asana (the way of sitting),
- ❧ mudra (the position of the hands),
- ❧ pranayam (a specified breath pattern), and
- ❧ mantra (a sound current, either audible or silent).

IMPORTANT GUIDELINES TO REMEMBER

1. Chant ONG NAMO GURU DEV NAMO (see page 180) at least three times before you start any Kundalini Yoga session.
2. Breathe only through the nose unless otherwise instructed.
3. You can cut down on the time of any exercise, but never increase it.
4. Relax at least thirty seconds and up to one minute after each exercise.

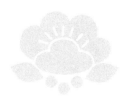

Kriya for Digestion

Yogi Bhajan taught this kriya to a gathering in Santa Fe, New Mexico, in July 1969,

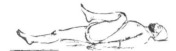

1. Lie on your back. Lift your legs twelve inches off the ground. Bend and straighten alternate legs in a push/pull motion, bringing each knee into the chest. Maintain the twelve-inch height as if your feet were sliding back and forth along a shelf twelve inches off the ground. (It is not a circular bicycle motion.)

Press your toes forward, and breathe deeply, synchronizing breath with movement.

Thirty seconds to one minute.

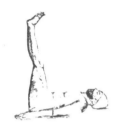

2. Lying on your back, keeping your heels together, lift both legs up ninety degrees as you inhale, and lower them as you exhale. Repeat this fairly rapidly for thirty seconds.

Rest and repeat for one minute. Rest again and repeat for thirty seconds.

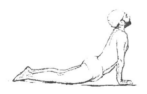

3. Turn over onto your stomach, put your hands under your shoulders, and come up into Cobra Pose. Bend your knees and strike your buttocks rapidly with alternate heels.

Thirty seconds to one minute.

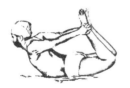

4. Catch hold of your ankles and stretch like a Bow, look toward the sky, and roll forward and back on your stomach, holding on to your ankles. (Try to keep the ankles together.) Thirty seconds to one minute.

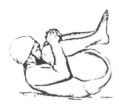

5. Lie on your back, bend your knees into your chest, clasping them with your arms, and roll forward and backward on your spine.
Thirty seconds to one minute.

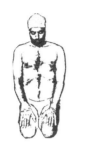

6. Sit on your heels in Rock Pose. Grab onto your heels from behind and bend forward to touch your forehead to the ground. (Make sure it's the forehead, not the top of the head.)
Hold the position up to one minute.

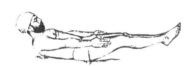

7. On your back, lift head and heels six inches from the ground; look at your toes. Do this Stretch Pose with Breath of Fire.
Try to maintain up to one minute.

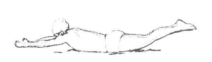

8. Boat Pose: Lie on your stomach, arms outstretched in front of you, fingers interlaced. Lift arms and legs up off the ground with arms hugging the ears.
Do with Breath of Fire for thirty seconds.

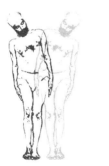

9. Stand up. Keep heels together. Swing slowly like a pendulum from side to side. Inhale up to center, and exhale as you lean sideways down to alternate sides. (Keep your arms relaxed at your sides and keep the motion sideways, not forward or back.)

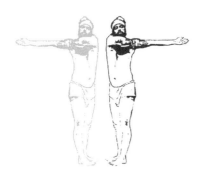
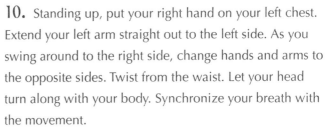

10. Standing up, put your right hand on your left chest. Extend your left arm straight out to the left side. As you swing around to the right side, change hands and arms to the opposite sides. Twist from the waist. Let your head turn along with your body. Synchronize your breath with the movement.
One or two minutes.

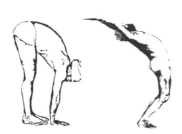

11. Standing up, keeping the knees straight but not locked, perform the Forward Bend: Touch your palms to the ground, then inhale and bring the arms up overhead (thumbs crossed over each other) and carefully lean back as far as possible without losing your balance. Hold the posture for a few seconds. (If you can't reach all the way forward and down, just reach as far as you can.)
Repeat ten or twenty times.

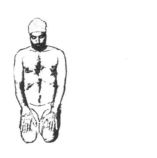

12. Sit on your heels in Rock Pose. Hold your hands in your lap in Venus Lock (fingers interlaced; see glossary). Let the breath be soft and normal, but regulated. Be aware of it flowing in and out. Meditate on your breath: in your mind hear SAT as you inhale, NAM as you exhale.
Five minutes.

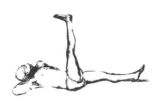

13. Lie on your back. Interlace your fingers under the back of your neck underneath your hair. On each inhalation raise one leg up, and on the exhalation, lower it back down. Continue alternating legs fairly rapidly.
Two minutes.

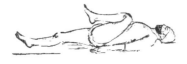

14. Lie on your back and repeat the first exercise (the push/pull motion of legs).
Thirty seconds to one minute.

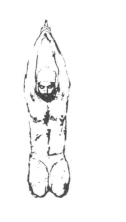

15. "Sat" Kriya: Sit on your heels and raise your arms overhead with the palms together, thumbs crossed. Chant SAT out loud as you pull in and up on the navel point and the sex organs and the rectum in the Root Lock (Mul Bandh); say NAM (softly) as you relax the lock. Continue for one or two minutes maximum, then inhale, exhale, and apply the Root Lock again, hold with the breath out for eight seconds, drawing the energy up the spine. Relax.

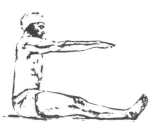

16. Sit with legs stretched straight out in front, arms out front parallel to the ground.
Perform the Breath of Fire in this posture for one minute.

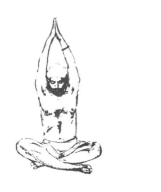

17. Easy Pose (Sukhasan): With your eyes closed, focus at the third eye point (between the eyebrows and up about one-eighth inch). Lift your arms up overhead, palms together, arms hugging the ears. Chant EK ONG KAR SAT NAM SIRI WAHE GURU (see page 182).
Two to five minutes.

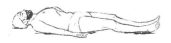

18. Enjoy Long Deep Relaxation in Corpse Pose.
Ten to fifteen minutes.

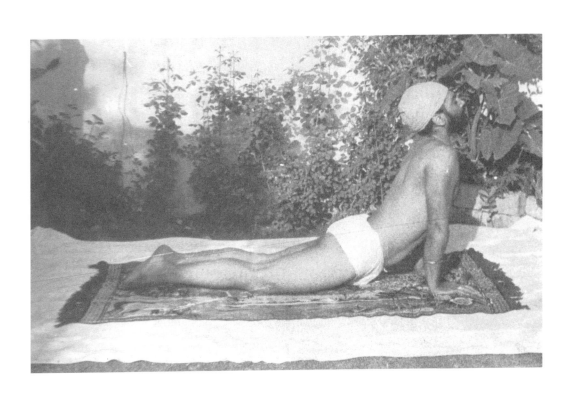

Cobra

BHUJANGASANA

SERPENT POSE

Your spine will be fine, stretch it up, please do.
Nerves and muscles tune up, of heart and abdomen too.
Develop your bust—with cobra you must
(It's what the yogis tell us to do.)

SPECIAL TIPS

Keep your fingers forward and elbows pressed into your sides, not spread out like wings. Ideal posture will be with straight arms and an expanded chest in front of your arms.[1]

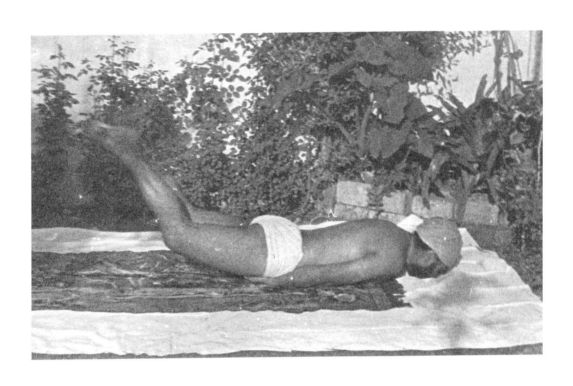

Locust

SHALAVASANA

Attention marathon walkers (and runners, too):
Locust builds up your stamina for whatever hard work or play you do.
Gets rid of rheumatism in hands, legs, and sciatic nerve.
To eliminate fat on your buttocks and hips, Locust also serves.
And for women there's extra benefit, a "bonus cure,"
No more pain at the sacrum when menses occur.

> Note: Avoid Locust if you have weak lungs, heart disease, hernia, peptic ulcer, or intestinal tuberculosis.

Good for Everything That Ails You

Yogi Bhajan taught this set when we were very new.
He called it: "Good for Everything That Ails You."
Three minutes each: Locust, Cobra, and Shoulder Stand
More than just postures, Kundalini adds action—
     Do it — if you can!

(A word of caution if you have weak lungs or heart disease:
Locust Posture is banned; practice some other set, please.)

Start with the Locust (of course you've tuned in,
We always, always tune in before we begin):
Three times vibrating ONG NAMO GURU DEV NAMO
Wise people chant to receive the flow
Of blessings, protection, guidance and power
Invoking Creator, Divine Teacher, opening each lotus flower.

How to do It

1. Locust Posture: Lie on your stomach, chin on the floor. Place your fists under your stomach near the hips. (My notes say, "It hurts.")

   Inhale and lift both legs up as high as possible. Keeping the legs up, exhale and apply the Root Lock, Mul Bandh (simultaneously contract the muscles of the rectum, sex organ, and navel point). Legs remain up throughout the exercise.

   Hold the position and hold the breath out as long as possible. When necessary, inhale, then exhale, and again apply the Mul Bandh, holding the breath out as long as you can each time. Continue this sequence for three minutes, continuing to hold the legs up throughout.

   > *Tip:* Locust is an extension exercise. In order to lengthen your spine, roll your hips and knees in toward each other. Otherwise, you just compress your lower back, and you want to be able to use the power of the back muscles to create the lift.[3]

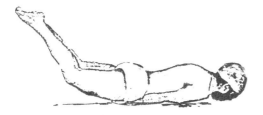

2. Relax on your back in Corpse Pose for two minutes.[4]

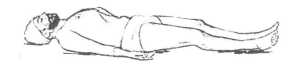

3. Cobra Pose: Lie on your stomach, chin on the floor, hands slightly under the outside of your shoulders, palms down, fingers pointing forward. Elbows are pulled in toward your ribs. Inhale and gently arch your upper torso as far as you can with ease. Then follow through by straightening your elbows, bringing up your chest. Pull your shoulders down and back, lifting your upper body high enough so that the pelvis comes slightly off the floor. That way your weight is on your hands, knees, and feet. The last thing to come into position is your head, which you tilt back—if your neck can support it, so that you can look at the ceiling, keeping your gaze fixed at one point. Try not to blink, even if your eyes water. Bend your elbows slightly to expand the chest; this will avoid putting pressure on your neck and lower back.

Inhale, exhale, and apply Mul Bandh. Repeat. Continue holding the pose, inhaling and exhaling, applying Mul Bandh on every exhalation, for three minutes.

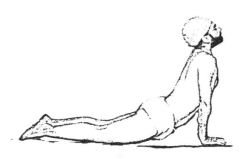

4. Relax on your stomach for two minutes. Turn your head to one side. Your arms can also be lying beside your body, hands toward feet, palms up.

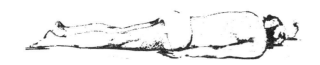

5. Shoulder Stand (WITH ACTION ADDED): (If necessary, review the description of the Shoulder Stand on pages 61–62.) Breathing only through the nose, inhale deeply, exhale, and hold the breath out while you begin rapidly kicking the buttocks with alternate heels. Keep kicking for as long as you can hold the breath out. Then immediately inhale as you lift the legs straight up. Exhale and begin kicking again. Continue this sequence for three minutes.

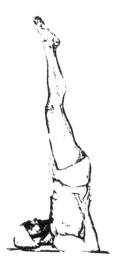

6. Relax in Corpse Pose at least two minutes.

Relaxation after each exercise is essential. It is just as important as the exercise itself!

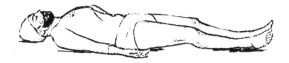

Spinal Trio

A complete spinal posture is formed
When you practice this trio as a daily norm.
The Cobra and Locust, along with the Bow—
Make a sincere effort to do them just so.
Strengthen the nerves and muscles of your entire spine—
Trio practiced correctly, will make you feel fine!

Two out of three postures you already know.
Simply you substitute—instead of Shoulder Stand: the Bow.
Mind you, this isn't a kriya, but a different style—
You just hold the postures for a little while.
There's no special movement or pranayam prescribed,
See if you experience the benefits the text described.

How to do It

WHEN YOU practice this trio of postures, Cobra, Locust, and Bow, inhale as you rise up into each posture and hold for a few seconds, then exhale as you relax down. Then repeat, coming up again, slowly. Inhaling up, exhaling down, breathing only through the nose, of course. You augment the power of the posture by mentally thinking SAT as you inhale, and NAM as you exhale. This Bij Mantra (seed sound) reaffirms your True (SAT) Identity (NAM).

For Locust, you may want to begin by lifting your legs alternately, one at a time (keeping them straight), and holding them up for not more than a few seconds. Then raise and lower both legs together, a maximum of five to seven times.

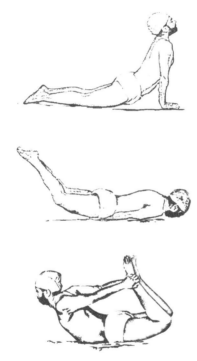

Remember, do not do Locust if you have heart trouble, weak lungs, hernia, peptic ulcer, or intestinal tuberculosis.

Super Excellent Set to Build Stamina

Yogi Bhajan first taught this energetic kriya in the summer of 1986, at Khalsa Women's Training Camp in New Mexico. He mentioned how valuable these exercises are; and in fact he taught it again in Los Angeles the following year.

IN THIS KRIYA, you chant HAR in rhythm with each beat of the exercise, moving from one position to the next without stopping (contrary to the usual relaxation after each exercise in most Kundalini Yoga kriyas).

"HAR" is one of the names of God. Chanting HAR specifically invokes the creativity of that one GOD who breathes in all of us. (GOD is that force, energy, intelligence, consciousness that Generates, Organizes, and then Delivers or Destroys everything, including you and me. How you choose to worship that one God is your religion.)

All of these exercises are done *standing up*. You will be activating the creative GOD in every cell of your body as you chant HAR with each beat.

Ordinarily, in Kundalini Yoga, we rest after each exercise, but this "aerobic" set is an exception to that rule. This is a nonstop tune-up!

Reason

- Crisscross jumping balances the metabolism.
- Archer Pose applies pressure on the thigh bone to balance calcium, magnesium, potassium, and sodium.
- Backward stretching works on the lymphatic system.
- Clapping the hands indirectly massages the brain.
- Pumping the arms stimulates the meridian points on the forearms to balance the colon, stomach, spleen, and liver.
- Stretching side to side moves the colon.

Glands are the guardians of your health. One of the great "secrets" of Kundalini Yoga, which accounts for its power and its dynamic and rapid results, is its ability to make the glands secrete. This comes from the way the kriyas are designed—creating pressure on the glands through specific angles of the body. Then relaxation allows the secretions that have been stimulated to circulate throughout the entire bloodstream, bringing balance to the entire system.

How to do It

HERE'S AN exception to the "relax after each exercise" rule! Go through the entire series without a break. Then relax.

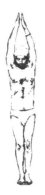

1. Standing with your feet together, clap your hands over your head eight times. Each time you clap, chant HAR with the tip of your tongue. (That means your tongue flicks the roof of your mouth, so the *r* is rolled—sounding almost like a *d*. And the *a* is short, sounding like the *u* in *butter*.)

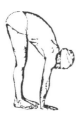

2. Bend over and pat the ground hard with both hands, eight times. With each pat, chant HAR with the tip of your tongue.

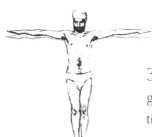

3. Straighten up with your arms out to the sides parallel to the ground. Raise and lower the arms one inch, patting the air eight times as you chant HAR with the tip of the tongue, eight times.

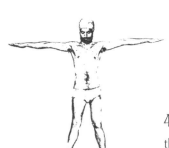

4. Jumping, crisscross the arms and legs, chanting HAR each time the arms and legs cross and each time they are out at the sides, for a total of eight HAR's.

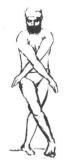

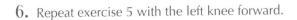

5. Do Archer Pose with the right leg forward. Bend the right knee, extending the stretch of the position eight times.

6. Repeat exercise 5 with the left knee forward.

7. Repeat exercise 4 (crisscross jumping and chanting).

KUNDALINI POSTURES AND POETRY

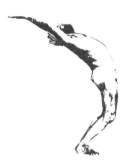

8. With the arms in the air over the head, lean backward eight times, chanting HAR with each backward bend.

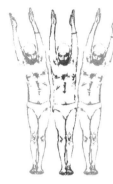

9. Repeat exercise 4 (crisscross jumping and chanting).

10. With the arms still over the head, bend to the left four times and then to the right four times.

11. Relax in Corpse Pose.

REPEAT THE SERIES

Five or six repetitions of this series will balance the entire body. Build it up to eleven minutes, then to thirty-one minutes or sixty-two. This kriya has so many positive effects that it stands out as one to practice regularly.

When you finish all the repetitions, be sure to relax long and deep in Corpse Pose. Corpse Pose is the best posture for optimum support for your spine. Lying flat on your back, be sure your body is in a straight line and that your hands are turned palms up.

Ten Bodies

Think you have just one body? Well, think again,
The fact of the matter is that you have ten!
What you see with the naked eye,
    made of bones and blood and tissue,
Your Physical Body, is just the visible layer
    of the many you were issued.

1.   Innermost and first is the Soul Body; it never dies,
     It's that reality/identity in you that people see
         when they look into your eyes.

2.   You don't have just one mind, count them, there are three:
     First is the Negative Mind to protect you
         by warning you where danger might be;

3.   Second is your Positive Mind which next comes into play
     Finding the benefits and values in whatever comes your way;

4.   Third, to ensure your conclusions/actions are wise,
     Your unbiased Neutral Mind should be used to decide.

5.   Already you've counted four bodies, now comes number five,
     The Physical Body you live in while you're alive.

6.   Sixth body, the Arcline, "halo," from ear-tip to ear-tip
         surrounds your head,

Silently projects (and protects) who you are,
  without a word being said.

7. Seventh is your Aura, the electromagnetic field (extending
    nine feet), an important shield that keeps you protected.
    By many who have special vision, it can be easily detected.

8. Your Pranic Body is fed with each inhalation,
      prolonging your life (it's number eight);
    Controls your breath, and when you keep it strong
      (through pranayam),
    You have courage, energy, power to heal,
      and strength to conquer your fate.

9. Ninth body is the most subtle, it carries your soul
      when you die.
    You can't see it, but the Subtle Body can see beneath
      the surface of the outer; reveals hidden meanings,
      makes you aware when people lie.

10. Your Radiant Body begins at the edge of the Aura,
    projecting spiritual royalty, radiance, and power;
    so then:
      All good things are drawn to you,
      through a well-developed number ten.

Through the perfection of each of the ten bodies,

the human psyche attains its wholeness.

This wholeness gives the human the protection it needs

to live fearlessly. . . . The purpose of conscious knowledge

that our ten bodies are working, is to produce the most

effective functioning human being, who can easily

deal with all of life's challenges.

—YOGI BHAJAN

Gifts of the Ten Bodies

Soul Body	gives	Humility
Negative Mind	gives	Obedience
Positive Mind	gives	Equality
Neutral Mind	gives	Service
Physical Body	gives	Self-Sacrifice
Arcline	gives	Justice
Aura	gives	Mercy
Pranic Body	gives	Purity
Subtle Body	gives	Calmness
Radiant Body	gives	Royal Courage

"Kundalini Yoga works on more than the Physical Body. In addition to the exercises, the use of the sound current (the recitation of shabd) is used. The tongue stimulates the eighty-four meridian points in the upper palate, for these specific sounds, chanted in certain combinations, cause the energy signal of the pineal gland to send an inward and outward combined signal to the cortex, as well as other functioning parts of the brain. These signals are transmitted through the neuro-message fluid. . . . One is then intuitively able to succeed in encounters with unfavorable circumstances, avoid unnecessary conflict, and remain strong and steady. Each shabd can repair one or more of our ten bodies."[5]

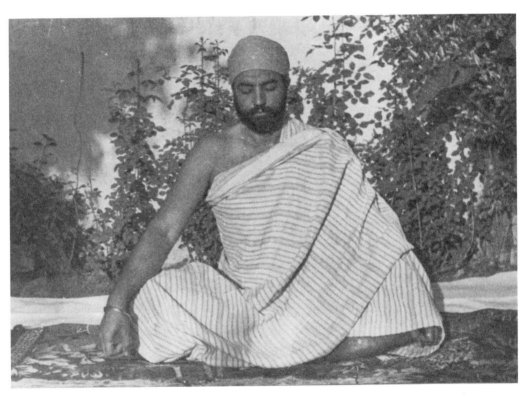

What does it mean to master a mantra?

When you have repeated it so much, so often and so well that you

hear it within you, and it comes handy to you—especially at the moment

of death—you have mastered a mantra.

—YOGI BHAJAN

10

SOUND ADVICE

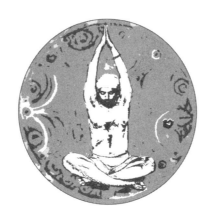

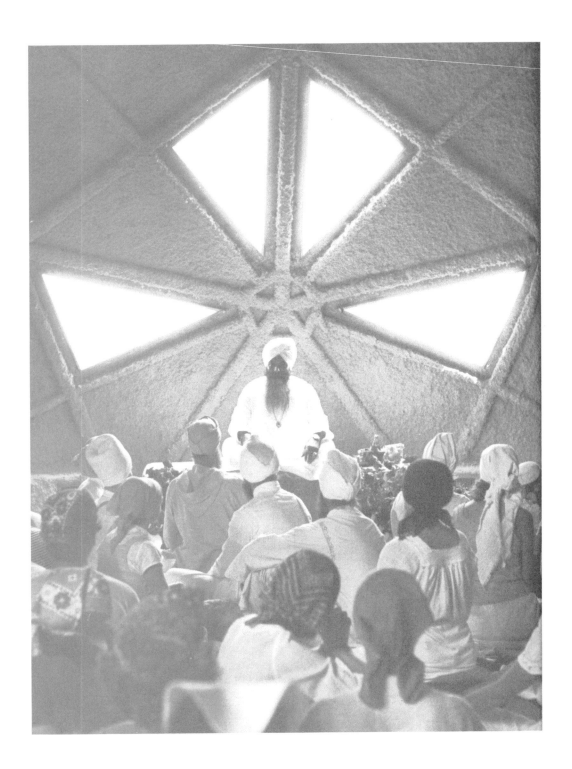

How to Chant

Basically, chanting is vibrating. It isn't speaking, it isn't singing (although we chant many mantras in various tunes). For most mantras, chant from the navel point; this is the point of power.

REASON

In the upper palate, there are eighty-four meridian points that are stimulated by the tip of the tongue when we chant. Different mantras create various patterns or combinations of sequential pressure on these meridian points, and these patterns activate the hypothalamus and in turn affect the pituitary. Thus an actual change takes place in the chemistry of the brain when we chant. Mantras are the "codes" to open the locks of awareness.

ONG NAMO GURU DEV NAMO

ONG NAMO GURU DEV NAMO is an invocation we use before starting any class or practice session of Kundalini Yoga. These syllables are the phone number connecting us to the Golden Chain of Consciousness of those masters who have preceded us on this path. When you want to watch a particular program on television or radio, you have to tune your set to the channel or station broadcasting the particular wavelength you want to receive. Similarly we chant to attune ourselves to the vibratory frequency of the consciousness we want to receive. In this case, we want to access the highest possible source of guidance, intelligence, and wisdom! So we call on the Creator and the Divine Teacher inside us.

Vibrating ONG summons the Creator. It is pronounced like the letter *o* with the *ng* added on. It should be vibrated at the back of the throat as the sound comes out through the nose.

NAMO offers "reverent greetings." Pronounce the *a* like the *a* in *above*, keeping it short in sound and duration. The *o* is just an *o*. The word *namo* is from the Sanscrit *nameste*. It implies humility and reverence for the giver of the divine teaching we are about to receive.

GURU is the giver of the technology. *Gu* means darkness, and *ru* means light. In other words, Guru is the one who dispels our ignorance. The GU syllable is very, very, very short and the RU syllable rhymes with *too*.

DEV is pronounced to rhyme somewhere between the sound of the name *Dave* and the *e* in the name *Ben*. When we say DEV, we are not calling on a person, but rather on the translucent, nonphysical consciousness of Guru. The invocation closes with reverence again, with NAMO. It is important always to chant this mantra at least three times before any Kundalini Yoga practice. And remember, chanting isn't singing, it isn't speaking, it is vibrating!

SAT NAM

SAT NAM rhymes with *but Mom*. The Bij Mantra (seed sound) SAT NAM means "Truth is your identity" and/or "God's Name is Truth."

180

Chanting SAT NAM reinforces the divine consciousness in everyone. You can use it as a greeting, anytime, anyplace. Put it on your answering machine. When you greet someone with "Sat nam" you are affirming the divine identity you both share—and for that moment you are truly one in the spirit. After that, if you must, you can argue about politics and religion; differ in your opinions and preferences in music, art, movies, clothing, and hairstyles—but at least for that first brief moment when you say "Sat nam," you have removed all barriers to soul-to-soul communication!

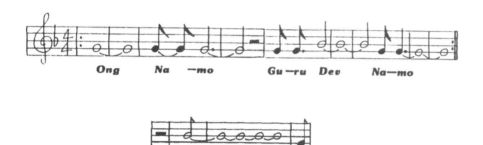

Ong   Na —mo   Gu —ru Dev   Na—mo

Sat . . . . Nam

ANG SANG WAHE GURU

ANG SANG WAHE GURU means that God is in every limb of my body.

WAHE GURU is a mantra of ecstasy; the words used to describe the indescribable, fantastic, wonderful, awesome magnificence of God.

Pronounce both the ANG and the SANG to rhyme with *sung*. WA is pronounced like the first syllable in *water*. HE sounds like *bay*. GURU is pronounced almost like one syllable, *groo*. The *u* is very, very short in GU, and the RU rhymes with *too*.

Ek Ong Kar Sat Nam Siri Wahe Guru

Long Ek Ong Kar's

Ek must be powerful, from the navel point strong,
Then (at the back of the throat—
    out through the nose—and not too long),
    powerfully vibrate the syllable ONG.
Slide directly into the KAR, no pause, no break so far,
Then inhale deeply and from your navel point chant SAT
    followed by NAAM—for that is what
To do before you reach for S'REE,
Then take in just a half breath and you will see
How easily you chant WA—then insert a tiny "hay"
Ending with G'ROO. To open all chakras, chant this mantra every day.

Please don't drop the tone between EK and ONG,
They have a relationship on the scale, where each belongs:
    ONG should not be lower than EK, please take care—
    Keep the pitch level—or higher—so the energy's there!

Remember, to make the kundalini flow,
ONG must not be too long, must not be too low!
From the back of the throat, out through the nose
Vibrate ONG properly, no one will doze!

EK from the navel point, also SAT and S'REE,
When chanted correctly, Ashtang Mantra can set you free!

"Mantram siddhyam, siddhyam parmesharam"—
    are you a doubting Thomas?
("He who masters mantra, becomes master of God,"
    the scriptures promise.)

Long EK ONG KAR's are designed to bring
Maximum power to those who can sing,
Vibrate, and chant with conscious control—
(In a group, this is the responsibility, the leader's role:
He or she has to chant powerfully, loud and clear
Keep the tempo "upbeat" and make sure everyone can hear.)

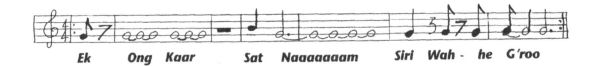

Ek　　Ong　Kaar　　Sat　Naaaaaaam　　Siri　Wah - he　G'roo

One Creator created this creation, Truth is His Name; He is so great we

have no words to describe His infinite, ultimate wisdom.

EK	One
ONG	Creator
KAR	Creation
SAT	Truth
NAM	Name (Identity)
SIRI	Great
WAHE	Beyond description—"Wow!"
GURU	Dispeller of darkness; or teacher

REASON

Mantram siddyam, siddyam paramesharam.

He who masters mantra, masters God Himself.

EK ONG KAR SAT NAM SIRI WAHE GURU was the first, and almost the only, mantra Yogi Bhajan taught us (except for SAT NAM and ONG NAMO GURU DEV NAMO) during his first year in the United States. It is extremely powerful and energizing. It opens all the chakras.

The ideal, most effective time of day to chant it is during what are called the "ambrosial hours," the two and one-half hours before sunrise in the morning. It is the first of seven mantras we chant in our morning sadhana. (Sadhana includes a total of sixty-two minutes of chanting.)

It has been said that a person can attain liberation by chanting this Ashtang Mantra correctly, for two and a half hours before sunrise for forty consecutive days. ("Correctly" would mean with full concentration.)

Other suggested time periods for your personal practice of this mantra are thirty-one minutes or one hour. Try it for yourself: "Doing is believing."[1]

How to do It

1. Be sure to apply the Neck Lock (pull your chin straight back).
2. Keep your spine straight.
3. Close your eyes.
4. Hold your hands in Gyan Mudra or Venus Lock (see glossary for descriptions).
5. Optionally, as you chant each syllable, you can concentrate on each chakra, from the first to the eighth.

Note: Mothers, this mantra is especially effective for you to chant, as you pray for your child.)

Morning and Night, Do It Right

❀

When you wake up in the morning
Do you feel sluggish, weird and wasted?
If so, try the 3HO bedtime routine,
Recipe for deep restful sleep, it's been yogically tested.
In the morning, awaken shiny and bright
Refreshed from a peaceful dreamless-sleep night

At least two hours before bedtime, finish your last meal and leave the table.
It's lovely to go for a walk before going to sleep if you're able.

Arrange your firm bed with head or feet placed east to west,
Protect your electromagnetic field, if you want to sleep best.
A little Kundalini Yoga to finish the day
Then wash your feet in cold water—that's the way
To get ready for a foot massage; aaaah so soothing and healing
At bedtime, it's oh so appealing.
Then put all your troubles on a shelf labeled "GOD."
Put on your CD or tape player, lie down ready for the land of Nod.

Begin long deep breathing on your stomach to start.
Close off your right nostril—this is a most important part—
Breathe only through left nostril because Ida[2] supplies

Cool, calm Moon energy—and because you're wise,

In a very few minutes you'll start to doze

Then turn on your back, if that's what you chose,

Or lie on your side if you prefer that position—

Make sure it's the right side, best for heart and digestion.

You can set your alarm clock if you must,

But also in your subconscious trust,

Tell it at bedtime what time you want to arise

And it will wake you—preferably before sunrise!

Yes, those ambrosial hours before the dawn appears

Are the ideal time for spiritual practice, proved through the years.

"Amrit Vela" (morning hours between four and seven)

Meditation is most effective at this time, to take you beyond even heaven.

When the time has come to arise

Follow this procedure, try it for size:

Keep your eyes closed, be kind to your nerves and don't just leap out of bed,

First take a few long deep breaths as you stretch your arms and legs.

Rub the palms of your hands together and the soles of your feet the same,

Then cover your closed eyes with the palms and slowly open your gaze.

Lift the hands slowly about eighteen inches high,

Protect your optic nerve from the shock of distance and light.

Bring your fingertips to your forehead, massage in a circular motion

Out to your temples and down to your chin, you don't need lotion.

Rub your nose, squeeze your ears; give yourself permission,

Waking up your face is part of this morning mission.

Stretch yourself left and right like a cat,

Breathing deeply of course, as you do that.

Still in bed, do Stretch Pose with Breath of Fire.

One minute or two adjusts your navel point and you won't be tired.

Then bend both knees up to your chest, lift your nose in between your knees,

Press for a minute with Breath of Fire then drop over on to your right side,
    if you please.

Knees still bent, lie for a moment—it's comfy and cozy—

Just don't fall asleep, if you start to get dozy.

Now get up gently, keep your feet bare

And walk to the bathroom, yogic routine continues there.

Brush the root of your tongue with powdered potassium alum and salt[3]

Till you almost gag and your eyes water, that's not a fault.

(Ancient teachings call that "cataract water" a boon for the eyes.)

Now comes the part that may be a surprise:

Before you step in the shower, massage your body with oil
(Almond oil recommended—scented or plain, you choose the style)
Then comes the challenge, the test of your mettle:
Turn on *cold* water only (for lukewarm don't settle).

Massage your body under cold water streaming,
Call on God if you feel like screaming!
ANG SANG WAHE GURU means "God is in every part of you"
So you can shout it—because it is true.

Cold water hitting your skin, blood rushes to the surface
   in self-defense,
Instantly improving circulation, opening capillaries,
   best hydrotherapy at no extra expense.
Dry off briskly with a rough towel till your skin glows—
What a great feeling, your body is happy from head to toes!

When you wake, tell yourself you are bountiful, blissful, and beautiful:

Bountiful—when you know your soul;

Blissful—neither pain nor pleasure affects you;

Beautiful—in adversity you speak the language of prosperity.

Do you think to give thanks for your arms and your legs? Your eyes

and ears? In those moments as you come out of the sleep state,

acknowledge how wonderful is this vehicle the Creator manufactured for

you to use during your visit to planet Earth.

—YOGI BHAJAN

Sadhana

Now you're ready to start your day by talking to your soul
"Sadhana"—your personal spiritual practice—helps you reach your goal.
Kundalini Yoga, chant, meditate, and sing.
Body and mind tuned up, enjoy every breath God will bring.

Any fool can sleep late and miss Sun's first rays
But blessed be the soul who wakes to the day
Two and a half hours before the Sun rises:
Best time for sadhana—practiced by the wisest.

Chant God's name before break of day
Sorrow and tension melt away
Sacred vibration in scientific combination
Stimulate hypothalamus, change brain cells' permutation.

Kundalini Yoga, meditation, and prayer
"Morning sadhana," your soul wants to be there.

(Excerpted from the poem "Sadhana" in *Kundalini Yoga: The Flow of Eternal Power*, p. 128.)

Seven Steps to Happiness

Those who seek happiness follow this rule:

(It can create wise men out of fools.)

Start with commitment, it's essential to win your life's goal,

Then character develops, bringing dignity,

so you can be whole;

Dignity brings out divinity, your natural state—

Which you can experience—with Guru's grace.

Finally, when you can sacrifice—and do it with a smile(!)

Your search for happiness has been worthwhile.

—YOGI BHAJAN

(The commitment is to your own higher consciousness; to consistency in your own practice, for your own benefit.)

11

AFTERWORDS

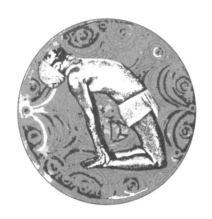

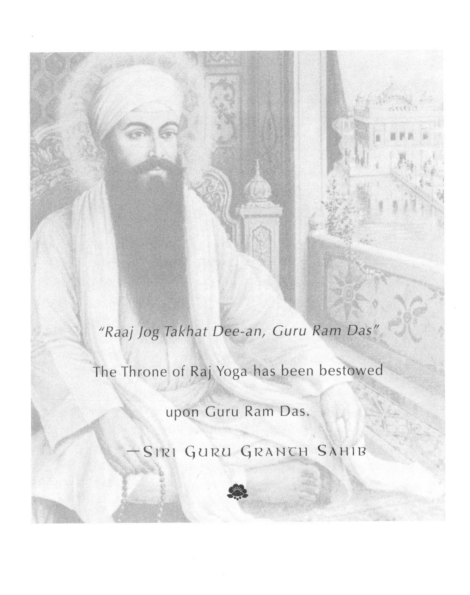

"Raaj Jog Takhat Dee-an, Guru Ram Das"

The Throne of Raj Yoga has been bestowed

upon Guru Ram Das.

—Siri Guru Granth Sahib

Yoga Traditions

NOWADAYS YOGA IS the "in" thing. Talk show hosts and celebrities endorse this or that yoga practice. It has been westernized and modernized to the hilt, and in some cases has been reduced to a physical workout, period. But authentic yoga of any path—whether it's Kundalini Yoga or Hatha, Karma, Bhakti or one of the many others—deals with the total being. The word *yoga* itself means to unite or "yoke" your individual consciousness with the universal consciousness. In other words, you become one with God. But please understand clearly, yoga is not a religion. When we speak of God in yoga, we mean the force, energy, or intelligence that Generates all creation, Organizes its creation, and then either Delivers or Destroys it. The way you worship that G-O-D is your religion. Yoga is, however, a sacred science, because it offers a method by which an individual can discover the divine Self, the G-O-D, within.

Traditionally in the East, to be allowed to learn Hatha Yoga, you would have had to take a vow of celibacy, live in solitude, give up all your worldly possessions, and totally devote yourself to your teacher and your practice. Such commitment would probably not appeal to most people flocking to health clubs and yoga studios throughout the world today.

Kundalini Yoga, on the other hand, demanded no such vows; however, it had its own requirements. Indeed, it was kept totally secret. Its practice was taught only to those few students who had proved their worth. They had to show consistent humility, obedience to the teacher, and self-discipline. The reason? Kundalini Yoga gives an individual great power. It was said that whoever taught it publicly "would not live to see his/her next birthday." But in 1969 Yogi Bhajan defied this warning, and began teaching openly—not only teaching Kundalini Yoga, but training students to

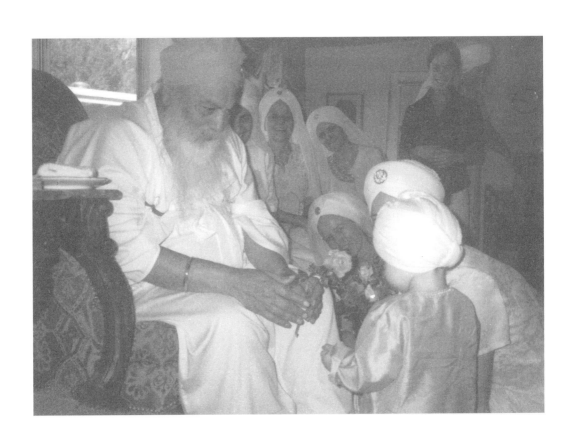

become teachers. He knew it was the method that would heal, uplift, and transform people most effectively, and he knew that people would soon be eagerly in need of a way to cope with the demands of the coming Aquarian Age.

Yogi Bhajan made Kundalini Yoga doable and accessible without diluting or polluting its sacredness. People found they could not only handle their normal daily lives more easily, but in fact thrive and prosper, becoming more competent and successful by investing a little time each day doing relatively simple kriyas.

ANCIENT HISTORY

To give you some idea of the intense dedication and qualifications it took to practice yoga in India in ancient times, here are some quotes:

In the classic *Bhagavad Gita*, Arjuna is instructed by Lord Krishna on how to control the mind through yoga:

> "The yogi should try constantly to concentrate his mind on the Supreme Self, remaining in solitude and alone, self-controlled, and relieved from desires and longings for possessions."

> "In a clean place which is neither too high nor too low and covered with the sacred grass, Kusa, a deer skin and a cloth, one over the other; sitting in asana, one must bring one's mind to concentrate, and controlling the thoughts and senses, one should practice the yoga of self-purification."

How about this?

> "By keeping the body, head, and neck erect and still, while looking fixedly at the tip of his nose, without allowing his eyes to wander, serene and fearless, firm in the vow of celibacy as well as in the thought of the Supreme Being, he should sit for the performance of yoga, with his mind turned to Me and intent on Me alone."

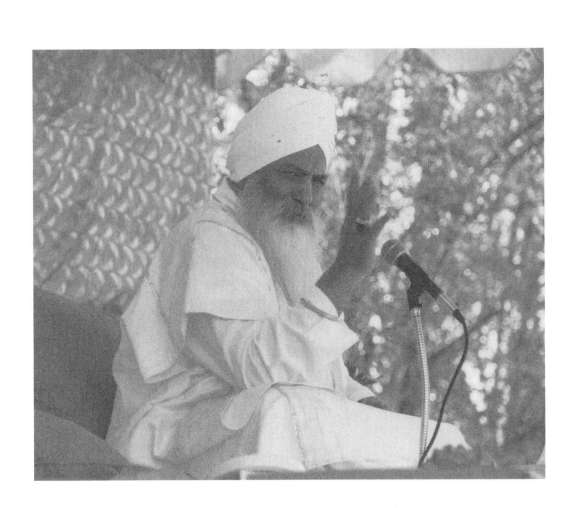

More practical instructions say (and these seem more applicable to current times):

1. Yogasanas are best performed at dawn, in the open air, but they can be done also at other times and near an open window.
2. The bowels must be cleared before starting the asanas. It is not desirable to bathe for two to three hours after the asanas, but a bath can be taken just before. No food or drink should be taken for four hours before starting.
3. The asanas must always be done barefooted on a carpet or rug spread out on a hard and even surface. Clothing should be as light and loose as possible.
4. It is not possible for those unaccustomed to the postures to do them correctly in the beginning, but through practice most of them can be mastered, particularly by young persons. Those in middle age should not strain to attain perfection in any of them. It should be possible without discomfort or pain.

And finally, the ultimate goal: Perfection:

"An individual is said to have perfected an asana when he can sit in that asana for a period of three hours and forty-eight minutes at a stretch."[1]

The postures you see in this book and the commentary are based upon the demanding traditional yoga that Yogi Bhajan mastered in India. He didn't require us to learn them all. In our Kundalini Yoga classes we practice only those that, in combination with breath and sound, most easily lead to greater awareness.

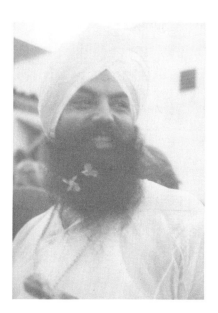

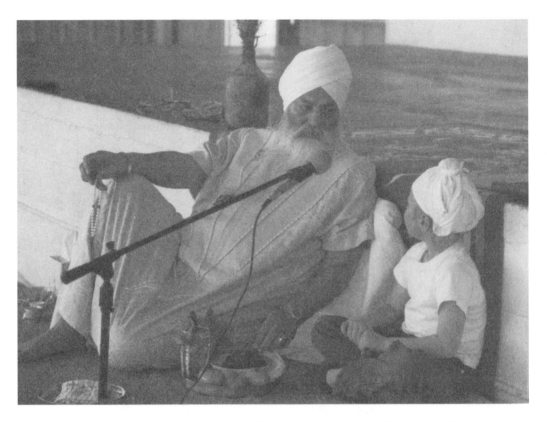

If you want to learn a thing, read that; if you want to know a thing, write

that; if you want to master a thing, teach that.

—YOGI BHAJAN

IKYTA

3HO formed a Kundalini Yoga Teachers Association,
 Established Teacher Training Courses with maximum participation

Reaching all over the world, IKYTA is truly international —
Practicing Kundalini Yoga has become quite fashionable.
No longer considered esoteric or strange in the West,
People have discovered teaching it—brings out your best.

IKYTA is pledged to maintaining the ethics and standards
 Yogi Bhajan brought;
Keeping the teachings pure, nothing added or subtracted,
Honoring everything the Master has taught.

Bibliography

Asana Pranayama Mudra Bandha
Swami Satyananda Saraswati
1969: Bhargava Bhusan Press, India

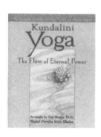

Kundalini Yoga: The Flow of Eternal Power
Shakti Parwha Kaur Khalsa
1998: Perigee Books, New York

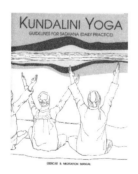

Kundalini Yoga: Guidelines for Sadhana (Daily Practice)
(Based on the teachings of Yogi Bhajan)
1996: Kundalini Research Institute, Pomona, California

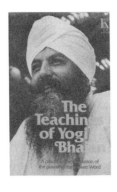

The Teachings of Yogi Bhajan
1977: Arcline Publications, Kundalini Research Institute, Pomona, California

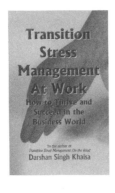

Transition Stress Management at Work:
How to Thrive and Succeed in the Business World
Darshan Singh Khalsa
2001: Lions Presence Press, Arizona

Yogasana Vijnana: The Science of Yoga
Dhirendra Brahmachari
1970: Asia Publishing House, India

Yogic Suksma Vyayama
Dhirendra Brahmachari
1965: The Caxton Press, New Delhi, India (in English)

Yogic Therapy: Yogic Way to Cure Diseases
Srimat Swami Sivananda Saraswati
1957: Swami Bijnanananda Saraswati, publisher
Umachal Prakashani
c/o Umachal Ashram
P.O. Kamakhya, Assam, India

Recommended Reading

Aquarian Times magazine
800-359-2940
siriram@kiit.com

Breathwalk
Yogi Bhajan, Ph.D., and Gurucharan Singh Khalsa, Ph.D.
Marvelous yogic technique for walking, meditation, and inner posture.
www.breathwalk.com <http://www.breathwalk.com>

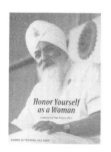

Honor Yourself as a Woman
(Lecture series by Yogi Bhajan)
Kundalini Research Institute
kri@newmexico.com
505-753-0562

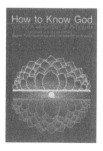

How to Know God: The Yoga Aphorisms of Patanjali
Swami Prabhavananda and Christopher Isherwood, translators
Vedanta Press, Hollywood, California

Sage of the Age
01-A Ram Das Guru Place, Espanola, NM 87532

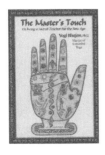

The Master's Touch: On Being a Sacred Teacher for the New Age
Yogi Bhajan, Ph.D.
Kundalini Research Institute, 1997

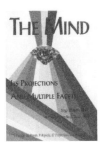

The Mind: Its Projections and Multiple Facets
Yogi Bhajan, Ph.D., with Gurucharan Singh Khalsa, Ph.D.
Kundalini Research Institute, 1998

Sources and Resources

3HO Foundation

888-346-2420
www.3ho.org
yogainfo@3ho.org

> Events include several yoga camps: the Summer and Winter Solstice Celebrations, KWTC (Women's Camp), and the International Peace Prayer Day Music Celebration (www.peaceprayerday.com).

IKYTA (3HO International Kundalini Yoga Teachers Association)

505-753-0423
505-753-5982 (fax)
www.kundaliniyoga.com

> Association of teachers in Kundalini Yoga and offers teacher training courses.

Kundalini Research Institute (KRI)

kri@newmexico.com

> (Look for this KRI seal of approval in any Kundalini Yoga book.)

Ancient Healing Ways Catalog

ahwc@kiit.com

> Offers books and music cassettes
> and CDs, as well as recorded lectures.

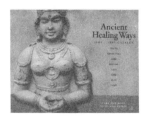

The Guru Ram Das Center for Medicine and Humanology

Shanti-Shanti Kaur Khalsa, Ph.D., director

P.O. Box 943

Santa Cruz, NM 87567

800-326-1322

www.grdcenter.com

healthnow@grdcenter.org

> Provides health education and instruction in yoga to persons with chronic or life-threatening illness and their family members.
>
> Training for health professionals to use these techniques in their practice and conduct research into the medical effects of Kundalini Yoga. Instructors utilize their training and experience in selecting kriyas and meditations that will best assist the individual in getting well.
>
> "We do not teach Kundalini Yoga to a diagnosis or a disease. We teach yoga to the person who has the disease. Kundalini Yoga is a sacred science. The sacredness of the client or student is awakened through it. Our clinical experience shows that a person who is ill can make a difference in their health recovery through the selective practice of Kundalini Yoga."
>
> —SHANTI SHANTI KAUR KHALSA, Ph.D.

Shakti Parwha Kaur Khalsa

P.O. Box 351149

Los Angeles, CA 90035

310-552-3416 ext. 14

sparwha@sbeglobal.net

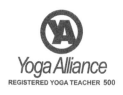

Yoga Alliance
REGISTERED YOGA TEACHER 500

Glossary

APANA	Outgoing, cleansing, or eliminating function of breath.
ASANA	Yogic posture—literally, "way of sitting."
ASHTANG	Eight.
BANDH	Lock: To direct the flow of energy, various "bandhs" or locks are applied by contracting specific internal muscles of the body. See also Mul Bandh, Jallunder Bandh, Uddhiyan Bandh. (Note: Venus Lock is a Mudra, not considered a Bandh)
BIJ MANTRA	Sat Nam is a Bij Mantra. Bij-seed. Mantra is a syllable or combination of syllables whose vibration has the inherent power to uplift consciousness.
BRAHMACHARYA	Renunciation and celibacy. The period of life—traditionally the first 25 years, after which a yogi may decide to take Brahmacharya vows—(not required on the Kundalini path), or marry and become a "householder," raising a family, for the next 25 years. From age 50 to 75 the wise yogi is to travel and share the acquired wisdom, and finally at age 75 settle down in one spot for the next 25 years (!) and disciples will come to learn from him!

CHAKRAS	Energy Centers. There are eight of these Projected Centers of Consciousness. Located at the: (the first five chakras are associated with the five elements.)

1. Rectum (to be more precise, perineum for men, cervix for women): Earth
2. Sex organs: Water
3. Navel Point: Fire
4. Center of Chest (heart chakra): Air
5. Throat: Ether
6. Center of forehead ("Third Eye point" or Ajna, or Agia Chakra) — Pituitary Gland
7. Top of the head ("Thousand Petalled Lotus" "Gate of Salvation" "Tenth Gate")
8. Aura: magnetic field that surrounds the body up to 9 feet in all directions. (Most texts only list the first seven chakras.)

Our consciousness, attitudes and behavior are directly related to the energy of the chakra from which we function at any given time.

DHARANA	Concentration: One of the steps on the Eight-fold path of Raj Yoga.
DHYAN	Meditation: One of the steps on the Eight-fold path of Raj Yoga.
GYAN MUDRA	*Gyan*, or *gian*, means "knowledge." Roll the index fingers just barely under the tips of the thumbs, so that the thumbs hold part of the nail; hold the other fingers straight and arms straight, no bend in elbows.

(When just tips of the thumbs and forefingers are touching, it is a "passive" Gyan Mudra, whereas the position described above is considered the "active" position, giving more control to the practitioner.)

IDA AND PINGALA	Ida is the name of one of the nerve channels carrying kundalini energy. It starts at the base of the spine, intertwines around the central column of the spine, and emerges in the left nostril. Pingala refers to the other nerve channel; it ends in the right nostril. Ida carries Moon energy; Pingala, Sun energy.
IKYTA	International Kundalini Yoga Teachers Association.
KARMA	A cosmic law of cause and effect: Action and reaction. "As you sow, so shall you reap." The actions we take create karma that we have to "pay." If not in this lifetime, in the next.
KRIYA	Completed action. A Kundalini Yoga exercise or series of exercises for a specific purpose. Usually combines mantra, mudra, asana and pranayam with movement.
KUNDALINI	"Spiritual energy." We already have kundalini energy coursing through our bodies carried in the two nerve channels of Ida and Pingala (which begin at the base of the spine and intertwine upward ending in the left and right nostrils). There is an extra reservoir, or dormant supply of kundalini energy under the fourth vertebra of the spine. Ideally, when it is awakened through the practice of Kundalini Yoga, it is allowed to travel up through the central column of the spine, the Shushmana, to activate the seventh chakra at the top of the skull.

"According to the physiology of Raja yoga, a huge reserve of spiritual energy situated at the base of the spine. This reserve of energy is known as the kundalini, 'that which is coiled up'; hence, it is sometimes referred to as the 'serpent power.' When the kundalini is aroused, it is said to travel up the spine through six centers of consciousness, reaching the seventh, the center of the brain."
(*How to Know God* p 112)

LOCK	*See* Bandh.
MANTRA	Sequence of syllables repeated silently or aloud.
MUDRA	Hand and arm position.
MUL BANDH	Also called Root Lock, this action closes off the first, second, and third projected energy centers of consciousness (chakras) so the kundalini energy can flow upward more easily. Muscles of the rectum, sex organ, and navel point are pulled in and up simultaneously. Mul Bandh can be applied after either an inhalation or an exhalation.
NECK LOCK	Chin is pulled straight back, straightening the back of the neck so the flow of kundalini energy is not blocked at the top of the spine. Also called Jallunder Bandh.
PATANJALI	The first yogi to ever write down what was known as the Eight Limbs (sometimes called "Steps") of Raj Yoga. Prior to his writing, all teaching of Raj Yoga was done verbally from master to disciple, and the disciple probably had to memorize the aphorisms, succinct statements that, of course, were explained in detail by the master. These aphorisms written by Patanjali have been translated to English. One of the best translations is by Swami Prabhavananda and Christopher Isherwood in the book *How to Know God*.
PRANA	Incoming "breath of life" received with each inhalation. The primary source of prana is the breath. Prana is also found in food and water, to greater or lesser degrees, depending upon the quality of the carrier. When the atom was split, the energy released was what the yogis have known for centuries as prana.
PRANAYAM	Yogic science of conscious controlled breathing.
PRATYAHAR	When the mind is in a state of absolute stillness (*shunya*), "zero." One of the steps on the Eight-fold path of Raj Yoga.

ROOT LOCK	*See* Mul Bandh.
SADHANA	Daily spiritual practice.
SHABD	Sound current. Often refers to sacred music.
THIRD EYE	Sixth chakra (*Ajna* chakra or *Agia* chakra). Allows one to "see the unseen"—it is the direct opening to intuition. Located between the eyebrows and up slightly about ⅛ inch. Focusing here for meditation activates the neutral mind and accesses intuition to receive the highest inner guidance and clarity.
UDDIYANA BANDH	This is the Diaphragm Lock. It is applied by lifting the diaphragm up high into the thorax and pulling the upper abdominal muscles back toward the spine, which should be straight. This creates a cavity that gives a gentle massage to the heart muscles. This lock is normally applied on the exhale. (Warning: Applied too forcefully on the inhale, it can create pressure in the eyes and heart.) This is considered to be a powerful lock since it allows the pranic force to transform through the central nerve channel of the spine up into the neck region. It also has a direct link to stimulating the hypothalamic-pituitary-adrenal axis in the brain. It stimulates the sense of compassion and can give a new youthfulness to the entire body.
VENUS LOCK 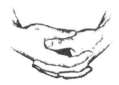	Hand position (mudra) that helps contain energy. Fingers are interlocked with thumb tips specifically applying slight pressure to the mound of Venus on one hand and the mound of Mars on the other. Right thumb tip of a male is pressed on the fleshy (Venus) mound of his left hand (between the left thumb and the wrist) while his left thumb tip is pressed in between the thumb and forefinger of his right hand (in the Mars "web"). Thumbs are not crossed, but lie side by side. Women reverse the hand position so that the left thumb

presses the fleshy mound of the right hand, and the right thumb tip is pressed into the web between the left thumb and forefinger. Then the other fingers are alternately interlaced, so that no two fingers of the same hand are next to each other. (Men's left little finger ends up on the outside, whereas women's right little finger ends up on the outside.)

YAMS AND NIYAMS "Don'ts and "Do's": Ethical precepts which a spiritual aspirant follows as guidelines for thought and action. The Yams and Niyams are the first steps on the eight-fold path of Raj Yoga as described in Patanjali's Aphorisms. (Translated in the book, *How To Know God*.)

YOGIC CLEANSING Specific methods of inner washing ("dhouti kriyas"), using water and air, have traditionally been employed by yogis to free the stomach, intestines and the abdomen of accumulated wastes or bacteria.

Notes

CHAPTER 1: Framing the Photos
   [1] See "Ten Bodies," p. 172.
   [2] Gurucharan Singh Khalsa, Ph.D.
   [3] "Truth is Your Identity"; Bij Mantra
   [4] See p. 179.
   [5] Yogi Bhajan

CHAPTER 2: Breath of Life
   [1] See "Ten Bodies," p. 172.
   [2] Sometimes called the "third eye," this energy center, the gateway to intuition, is related to the pituitary gland.

CHAPTER 3: Day by Day in the Correct Way
   [1] Gurucharan Singh Khalsa, Ph.D.
   [2] Gurucharan Singh Khalsa, Ph.D.
   [3] *Yogic Suksma Vyama*, pp. 143, 144 (Slokas Nos. 13–16—Yoga-Cudamany Upanishad, Part I).
   [4] *Yogic Suksma Vyama*, p. 161.
   [5] Guru Prem Singh Khalsa.
   [6] *Yogic Therapy*, p. 409.
   [7] *Yogasana Vijnana* (p. 49) advises: "Heels must touch each other while the toes point outwards."

[8] Guru Prem Singh Khalsa.

[9] Gurucharan Singh Khalsa, Ph.D.

[10] *Yogic Therapy*, p. 47.

CHAPTER 4: Stretching the Spine

[1] Guru Prem Singh Khalsa.

[2] Guru Prem Singh Khalsa.

[3] Guru Prem Singh Khalsa.

[4] *Yogic Therapy*, p. 334.

CHAPTER 5: Animal Nature

[1] *Prana* and *apana*—see glossary.

[2] *Chakras*—see glossary.

[3] *Yogic Therapy*, p. 377.

[4] Guru Prem Singh Khalsa.

CHAPTER 6: All Bent Into Shape

[1] Diaphragm Lock—see *bhand* in glossary.

CHAPTER 7: Standing Up Right!

[1] From "Trees" by Joyce Kilmer.

[2] Yogi Bhajan

[3] Guru Prem Singh Khalsa.

[4] Guru Prem Singh Khalsa.

CHAPTER 8: Meditation Postures

[1] Guru Prem Singh Khalsa.

[2] *Yogasana Vijnana*, p. 16.

[3] Guru Prem Singh Khalsa.

CHAPTER 9: Kundalini Yoga Kriyas

[1] Guru Prem Singh Khalsa.

[2] See page 180.

[3] Guru Prem Singh Khalsa.

[4] Yogi Bhajan

[5] Yogi Bhajan

CHAPTER 10: Sound Advice

[1] Yogi Bhajan.

[2] See *Ida and Pingala* in glossary.

[3] Use two parts powdered potassium alum and one part salt on your wet tooth-brush: brush the root of your tongue several times. Spit out—and get rid of the bacteria that have accumulated overnight.

CHAPTER 11: Afterwords

[1] *Yogasana Vijnana*, p. 4.

About the Author

[1] CD: www.spiritvoyage.com.

Index

222

About the Author

KNOWN AS the Mother of 3HO, Shakti Parwha Kaur Khalsa was the first woman in the United States to be trained in Kundalini Yoga by the Master, Yogi Bhajan. She has been teaching since 1969. Author of *Kundalini Yoga: The Flow of Eternal Power*, her modern, reader-friendly style has made this ancient sacred science easy and appealing to both new students and seasoned practitioners. She created a "Tool Kit for Teaching Beginners Kundalini Yoga," which is used in all KRI teacher training courses. For over thirty years she produced the 3HO newsletter, *The Science of Keeping Up*. Shakti edits the IKYTA *Kundalini Rising* and *Prosperity Paths* newsletters and is a contributing editor for *Aquarian Times* magazine.

Born in 1929 in Minneapolis, Minnesota, Shakti lives in Los Angeles, California, where she teaches beginners Kundalini Yoga, facilitates White Tantric Yoga courses, and continues to work on publishing the teachings of Yogi Bhajan. Certified by IKYTA and a member of the Yoga Alliance, she was ordained as a minister of Sikh Dharma in 1973.

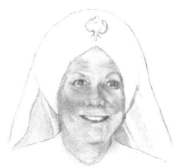

Shakti is an avid moviegoer, known for her youthful exuberance, lighthearted humor, and tendency to burst into song. She recorded her first CD, *Lord of Miracles*, in 2002.[1]

Credits

Photos on pages 12, 43, 46, 48, 52, 54, 60, 64, 66, 68, 70, 72, 74, 76, 78, 80, 82, 84, 86, 88, 90, 92, 94, 96, 100, 102, 104, 106, 108, 110, 114, 116, 118, 120, 122, 124, 126, 128, 132, 135, 136, 138, 140, 142, 144, 146, 148, 150, 158, 160, 190 courtesy Yogi Bhajan.

Photos on pages xv, 22, 31, 57, 152, 178, 199 by Satsimran Kaur.

Photos on pages 41, 196 courtesy Shakti Parwha Kaur Khalsa.

Photos on pages 2, 10, 18, 24, 28, 32, 34, 38, 112, 130, 148 by Lisa Law.

Photos on pages 198, 200 by Naryan Singh Khalsa (Phoenix, AZ).

Photos on page 8 courtesy of the *Los Angeles Times* (circa 1969).

Photos on pages 36, 194 from *The Man Called Siri Singh Sahib*. Reprinted with permission.

Photo on Page 4 courtesy of 3HO Foundation.

Photos on pages 174, 176 taken in Russia by an unknown photographer.